DON'T
YOUR GUIDE TO LIVING WELL
BACK
WITH A SPINAL CORD INJURY
DOWN

Derek Jones PhD, MBA

Rethink

First published in Great Britain in 2022
by Rethink Press (www.rethinkpress.com)

© Copyright Derek Jones

All rights reserved. No part of this publication may be reproduced, stored in or introduced into a retrieval system, or transmitted, in any form, or by any means (electronic, mechanical, photocopying, recording or otherwise) without the prior written permission of the publisher.

The right of Derek Jones to be identified as the author of this work has been asserted by him in accordance with the Copyright, Designs and Patents Act 1988.

This book is sold subject to the condition that it shall not, by way of trade or otherwise, be lent, resold, hired out, or otherwise circulated without the publisher's prior consent in any form of binding or cover other than that in which it is published and without a similar condition including this condition being imposed on the subsequent purchaser.

Cover image licensed by Ingram Image

Illustration on p58 © alekseymartynov | Adobe Stock

Author's disclaimer

Consider all information in this book to be general guidance offered in good faith to be used at your own risk. This material does not constitute personalised advice and is not intended to replace or substitute advice from a relevant professional who knows your personal circumstances.

Throughout the book, I mention some unique products that Anatomical Concepts deals with. I suggest reviewing alternatives to the ones I mention, if these exist. There are no 'perfect' products that will always be suitable for every individual, so the fact that I mention a product should not be considered a personal recommendation.

To my wife, Sandra, and children, Stephen and Carolyn

Contents

Introduction	1
PART ONE The Beginning	9
1 The Nature Of A Spinal Cord Injury	11
Spinal cord injury statistics	12
What happens at the time of injury?	16
Classifying an injury	18
Summary	25
The Christopher Reeve story	27
2 The Evolution Of Treatment	31
The emergence of specialist care	32
The first spinal-injury units	35
Sir Ludwig Guttmann	36
The democratisation of healthcare	40
Summary	44
Mark Pollock's story	45

3	**Assorted Mind Games**	**49**
	Being realistic	50
	A better you	53
	Three principles	57
	The power of the heart	61
	Techniques for resourcefulness	66
	Attitudes and beliefs	74
	Summary	80
	Claire Lomas's story	**82**
4	**The Rehabilitation Journey**	**85**
	Injury and negligence	86
	The home environment	87
	The charity sector	90
	The purpose of rehabilitation	93
	Neuroplasticity	97
	Goal setting in rehabilitation	103
	Summary	105
	Dan Eley's story	**107**
PART TWO Long-term Health		**109**
5	**Fit For Life**	**111**
	Exercise is medicine	112
	Standing for health	115

A low-cost alternative	124
Intensive rehabilitation centres	126
Training and exercise	129
Nutrition following injury	137
Summary	147
Joe English's story	**148**
6 Technology	**151**
Regaining or enhancing walking function	152
Orthotic bracing	157
Exoskeletons	163
Electrical stimulation	169
FES cycling	179
Electrical stimulation of denervated muscle	185
Electrotherapy and pain	189
Transcutaneous spinal cord stimulation	192
Assistive technology	194
Summary	196
7 Research Trends	**199**
Neuroprotection	202
Repair and regeneration	204
Cell-based therapies	206

    Retraining central nervous system circuits   208
    Summary   209

Final Thoughts   **211**
    Next moves   213

Glossary   **215**

Bibliography   **221**

Organisations   **235**

Acknowledgements   **237**

The Author   **241**

Introduction

'Spinal injury is a battle, a struggle. I don't want to stay like this. I want to walk ... I'll keep going until a cure is found.'
— Richard (disabled through sport)

Think about this quote for a moment. What does it take to live well following a spinal cord injury? Is it a case of just accepting your disability and moving on emotionally or, like Richard, do you grasp that it's another of life's challenges to face – one you can at least try to overcome?

Some people think that having a disability is an insurmountable barrier to quality of life. You must think differently if you want your life back on track.

The mindset, attitudes and beliefs of the injured person and those around them will have a great impact on their potential for recovery, but there are limits to how far 'belief' will take them. Just believing that something is possible is not enough to make it so. None of us can defy gravity and flap our arms to fly, however much we may believe we can. In my own business and professional life, I have come to understand the importance of adjusting my mindset – mental and emotional state – to overcome fear of failure. This knowledge is essential for anyone who wishes to succeed at anything – including overcoming a disability.

One of the great privileges of working with spinal cord injured people is I get to see how human ingenuity and spirit combined with know-how can lead to results that seem super-human. Barriers will always exist, but restoring a person's quality of life is more often limited by the resources, structures and processes of health and social services than it is by any lack of knowledge of rehabilitation.

In the UK, the National Health Service (NHS) finds it difficult, if not impossible, to deliver comprehensive lifelong physical rehabilitation to people following a catastrophic injury. The NHS is great at providing the vital medical care you need after injury, but rehabilitation can mean a long and daunting journey, so I advise you to choose to take some control over what that means. If you are injured, you must take responsibility for your rehabilitation. There are deep reasons for this, but briefly, it's about the need for control we all have as humans. Without some control, we set ourselves up to feel helpless.

INTRODUCTION

No healthcare system in the world will be able to meet all your needs and wants for your lifetime. Once your acute treatment is over and rehabilitation starts, it is very much like managing a complex project to achieve a goal, coordinate a military campaign or build a business. Even setting a goal won't be easy. You might know what you would like to happen, but it's often difficult to know if this is possible. Even if it is, you will need the mindset to keep going despite inevitable difficulties. It's certainly not about setting audacious goals – they will set you up for failure.

A key message I would like you to take from this book is that more recovery is possible than you may initially dare to hope. No one is promising a full physical recovery, but that does not close the door on you having a satisfying and meaningful life. You can set realistic goals and make plans to reach them. You can learn from others, share what you learn and develop attitudes and beliefs that serve you rather than limit you. In the resources section at the end of the book, you will find a link to bonus material which I will continue to refine based on the feedback I receive from you and other readers. As you go through the book, you will find some key points which are important too.

As I'm sure is clear by now, I have written this book with spinal cord injured people in mind – perhaps this relates to you or someone you care about. This is not a medical textbook or a comprehensive guide to all aspects of rehabilitation in spinal cord injury. What I aim to provide is some guidance and insight to make it easier for you to get your life back on track, drawing on a long experience of working with spinal cord injured clients and supplying technology and services for a range of assistive and therapy situations.

This book will sketch out a rough 'map of the territory' and provide information on issues that you will need to confront. Together, we will look at proven technologies and emerging research and developments that may impact your potential for recovery and long-term health. You will find references to scientific literature, which the more enthusiastic among you can look up for further information, and a glossary at the end of the book will define specialist terms for you.

Misinformation and lack of knowledge lead to all manner of problems. All too often, people leave hospital and buy various pieces of equipment without a guiding plan or knowledge of what is possible. It's too easy to believe that the latest technology will help (and yes, it might), then wake up one day to find your house full of equipment that neither works well together nor helps you meet your goals or expectations. To avoid these problems, you need to seek guidance you can trust and develop a realistic plan.

People can get excited about new technology, but some of the most effective technologies, such as electrotherapy and methods of exercise, have been around for a long time. Despite this, they are still not always well understood by clinicians, so it is hard for their patients to expect to benefit from their application. By sharing the stories of some of the amazing individuals

I have met, I will show you that, with the help of these and other technologies, a spinal cord injury does not mean that your life moving forward can't be fulfilling.

What to expect from this book

Don't Back Down is organised into two parts that represent stages in the life journey after a spinal cord injury: 'The Beginning' and 'Long-term Health'. To see how far things have progressed, we often need to start by looking back in time. In Part One, we will look at the nature of a spinal cord injury as well as the origins of treatment and the related care. We will look at topics such as mindset, stress and emotion, the reason being that they are important, even vital, to how we make decisions and the outcomes we experience in life.

We all need resilience to make our way through life, but this is much less about 'toughing it out' than people may think. No one who has a spinal cord injury should ever be blamed for having high expectations of recovery; too often, though, they don't receive the physical and emotional support to maximise the possibilities for that recovery. Developing inner resilience is the only way.

I want great outcomes for everyone. An individual's 'state' (a bundle of what they think and feel) determines what behaviours are possible for them and, of course, these behaviours shape their results in life. You can take someone with a spinal cord injury and provide excellent know-how and technology to help them with physical recovery, but it is always the individual's mindset that amplifies what they can achieve. Without a resilience mindset, any action they take is lacking in power.

We will look at the essence of rehabilitation and what it aims to achieve, and consider what happens with medico-legal cases when injury comes about due to another party's negligence. This may not be your personal situation, but nevertheless, there are valuable lessons you can learn about how rehabilitation is managed in these cases. We will also look at how best to adapt your home to your new needs and take a glimpse at how the charity sector may be able to help you.

Neuroplasticity is a term that I often hear these days to indicate the process that the human body can use to recover from trauma. It has brought hope that more recovery is possible than we may previously have believed. In Part One, we will explore what neuroplasticity means and what it suggests about how technology and training can help to carry out goal setting in rehabilitation.

In Part Two, we will consider some of the approaches and technologies that are being used to promote long-term health and functional recovery for people with a spinal cord injury. Perhaps the oldest and most practical 'technology for health' is exercise, and this is something that everyone needs. Whatever the level of injury, exercise is medicine, and we will look at how best to get it. We'll consider the recent trend to open private intensive-therapy centres and

INTRODUCTION

draw some comparisons with the world of strength and conditioning training to give you guidance on how to train.

Not everyone is blessed with the funds to attend a specialist-therapy centre, so how do you train for functional progress when money is tight? Part Two will look at functional electrical stimulation (FES) cycling and exoskeletons, along with orthotic bracing and other therapy and assistive technology.

We will also examine nutrition. Alongside exercise, nutrition is vital for health, but it can be complex and confusing. Finally, we'll look at emerging research that shows promise in pushing back the frontiers of knowledge of spinal cord injuries.

Now you know what to expect from the book, it's time to look forward to being the best version of yourself in the future. What better place to start than at 'The Beginning'?

PART ONE
THE BEGINNING

In this part, we will look at some basic information about spinal cord injuries and how treatment has progressed over the years. The spinal cord connects to the brain at the brain stem, and then runs right down to the lower back through the bony spinal column. It consists of nerve bundles and cells that carry 'messages' to and from the limbs and all parts of the body. A spinal cord injury disrupts these messages with serious consequences.

A catastrophic injury doesn't just affect the body, though; it shakes up our attitudes and beliefs about what might be possible for us in the future. For all of us, this shock results in feelings of loss of control. Our path through life, which was once so clear, is now filled with uncertainty. Research evidence suggests that the desire to have some control and make choices is vital to our survival (Magness, 2022). This desire is not something we have learned but seems to be 'wired in' as part of our biological drive.

Some individuals seem to adapt their mindset effortlessly to their situation and aim to rise above it. Others feel their apparent loss of control more deeply and struggle to adjust to the challenge. We will consider attitudes, beliefs and mindset and some of the resilience techniques we can use to get life back on track.

ONE
The Nature Of A Spinal Cord Injury

The spinal cord is situated within the protective bony spine, which consists of a series of vertebral segments that are described as cervical (neck area), thoracic (mid-back), lumbar (low back) and sacral (low back at the pelvis). The spinal cord itself also has so-called 'neurological' segmental levels which are defined by the spinal roots that enter and exit the spinal column between each of the vertebral segments. The spinal cord segmental levels do not necessarily correspond to the bony segments.

When people are injured, they are often told that they have damage to particular bony vertebrae and the cord itself at a given level, along with a further qualifier suggesting the severity of injury, ie 'complete' or 'incomplete'. The original grading system used to classify injuries was the Frankel classification (Frankel et al 1969). This was improved over time and the grading system commonly used now is the American Spinal Injury Association system (ASIA, 1982).

We will look in more depth into the level and location of a spinal cord injury and why this matters later in the chapter. First, though, let's examine some data.

Spinal cord injury statistics

If you have a spinal cord injury, you may wonder why you should bother about statistics. After all, you have become the 'statistic', but these insights shape the attitude of public and private sector policy makers, who in turn dictate the level of investment in products and services to help people like you. Far more people get injured each year in the UK, for example, than was previously thought, which is important knowledge as public spending tends to be influenced by the number of people affected.

Stop and think for a moment about whom you would expect to get injured and how. Are they likely to be young or old? What about what they will be doing at the time of the injury? I have found it hard to see an overall pattern – I have clients who have fallen from horses, bikes, scaffolding, a kitchen stool and even from bed. Oh – and by the way, always advise your family members to hold the handrail when on the stairs.

Many of today's injured individuals will not necessarily match the commonly held conception that a

THE NATURE OF A SPINAL CORD INJURY

younger person is more likely to have a spinal cord injury; they will often be older people, injured because of falls in the home. Many older folk remain active and perhaps provoke nature's sense of humour a bit. The mean age at injury has increased from 28.3 years in the 1970s to 37.1 years in 2005–2008 and the age profile is expected to rise further as the general population ages (DeVivo and Chen, 2011).

More people are being diagnosed with an illness or condition that results in paralysis and more women are sustaining an injury. The research shows that spinal cord injury occurs three to four times more often among males than females, but the proportion of injured females is rising as the population ages. Also, as we will see later in this chapter, the location of the injury matters when it comes to recovery and approximately half of all injuries are at the cervical part of the spine.

Lack of available resource will mean that, despite the well-established tried-and-tested care regimes that exist in regional spinal-injury units, many people will not be able to access this specialist care in a timely fashion – if at all. Recent studies have revealed more about the true economic costs of injury and how the specific nature of that injury affects these costs. In an ideal world, everyone with a spinal cord injury would receive all the care and support they need and want for a lifetime. This is not realistic, but knowing the true economic impact can help us make the case for improved measures to prevent such injuries as well as gain support from policy makers for those affected and needing support.

Despite the importance of economic evidence in health policymaking, there have been few estimates of true costs. In the UK, the National Institute for Health and Care Excellence (NICE) guidelines (NICE, 2016) relied on an expert opinion estimate of £2.5 million in average lifetime costs for spinal injury, with costs ranging up to £10 million. A more recent study estimated the direct and indirect lifetime costs from initial hospitalisation of all expected new traumatic and non-traumatic spinal cord injuries over twelve months (McDaid et al, 2019). The authors found that lifetime costs for an expected 1,270 new cases per annum were conservatively estimated as £1.43 billion in 2016 prices. They estimated a mean of £1.12 million (median £0.72 million) per case, ranging from £0.47 million to £1.87 million depending on the severity of injury. Potentially, 71% of lifetime costs 'are paid by the public purse with remaining costs due to reduced employment and carer time'.

Spinal cord injury statistics have not been especially easy to obtain in the past. For decades, the 'rule of thumb' for the UK was to expect around 1,000 new cases per year. New data, thanks to improved reporting from the eight specialist centres in England (SCI Annual Statement 2018/19), suggests that this figure was a gross underestimate.

The Scottish Spinal Injury Unit (QENSIU, 2021) supports the smaller population in Scotland compared to England and reported 103 new admissions in 2020/21; a reduction of thirty-six compared with the previous year, probably due to the pandemic restricting public activity. The total population living with such injuries in the UK has also been revised up to 50,000 from 40,000 (SCI Annual Statement 2018/19).

Medical advances mean that life expectancy for people living with a spinal cord injury is now broadly the same as for non-injured people. This implies that the total number of people living with a spinal cord injury will continue to grow. Unfortunately, research indicates that only between one-third and half of recently injured people can access specialist NHS care via the dedicated spinal-injury units and those who do so can expect lengthy delays prior to admission. Charities associated with the condition are calling for the government to resource this area appropriately. Everyone involved must develop a better understanding of the needs of people who have been paralysed by a spinal cord injury.

KEY POINT

The number of people being injured or diagnosed each year in the UK with a spinal cord injury is now around 2,500 – some thirty-five per week. The total number of people living with an injury in the UK is estimated to be 50,000, but it's likely that not all of these people will be able to access a spinal-injury unit.

If you do access one, you will have to get to work on your rehabilitation if you want to remain in the unit. Rehabilitation is not something done to you – you will be an active participant.

What happens at the time of injury?

People who sustain a spinal cord injury require urgent specialised care. It's not just a matter of survival; the nature of the immediate care has major implications for the individual's avoidance of complications and prospects for the long term. Complications damage their prospects for recovery and can have profound effects for the individual and society in general.

I'm going to talk as if all injuries are due to trauma. Of course, this is not always the case; there can be other medical and surgical causes, but it makes presenting the material a bit clearer and fundamentally, the consequences are largely similar.

Basically, all major trauma networks should have a defined link to a specialised spinal-injury unit and follow established protocols. We won't delve too deeply into all aspects of acute care here, but the interested reader can access publications by the National Spinal Cord Injury Strategy Board (NSCISB, 2012) or the guidelines by NICE (2016).

The timeline of a spinal cord injury caused by trauma is often described as consisting of a primary and a secondary phase. The primary phase is obviously mechanical – mainly due to the trauma to the spinal column, which in turn exerts force on the spinal cord it surrounds, resulting in disruption of axons (nerve fibre) (Rowland et al, 2008). This is most commonly the result of a compressive/bruising injury that causes shearing, laceration or acute stretching of the cord.

THE NATURE OF A SPINAL CORD INJURY

Injuries that fully cut through the spinal cord are rare and usually some connections are spared. These are 'incomplete injuries', as we will learn shortly. This seems to suggest that some functional recovery should be possible and research is ongoing for potential therapies that would optimise such recovery, which means at least preserving and developing the remaining connections. However, these remaining connections are at risk during the secondary phase of injury.

This phase features processes that the body initiates naturally as part of its inflammatory and healing response, but these processes – namely ischemia, excitotoxicity, cardiovascular dysfunction, oxidative stress and inflammation that leads to cell death (Rowland et al, 2008) – are damaging to the potential for recovery. At work, they are often harmful to the surviving neurons, and damage to these neurons can lead to poor functional recovery (Vawda and Fehlings, 2013).

During this secondary phase, an internal environment is created that impairs the potential for regeneration. The secondary phase is made up of several sub-phases that are divided over time into the so-called immediate (first two hours), acute (two to forty-eight hours), subacute (forty-eight hours to fourteen days), intermediate (fourteen days to six months) and chronic (six months and beyond) stages of injury. Typically, early therapy is designed to target the events that occur in a particular phase.

New neuroprotective, neuroregenerative and cell therapies are under investigation, with many already in clinical trials. Strategies that promote neuroregeneration after spinal cord injury recognise that there is injury to the axons and demyelination which damages the function of a nerve. The death of neurons results in cyst formation and something called 'glial scarring', which, again, is a part of the natural healing process that results in damage to the potential recovery, in this case, the formation of a physical and chemical barrier to regeneration.

The ideal treatment has a multifaceted approach to target the multiple processes arising in this type of injury which have the greatest impact on future patient outcomes and quality of life. As always, it is much easier to prevent conditions arising than to deal with them later in rehabilitation. There is often some functional recovery as part of the healing process, but the nature and extent of this varies.

KEY POINT

Injuries that fully cut through the spinal cord are rare, but this is not always recognised by patients. Early treatment will vary with the time since injury and is characterised by preventing complications that will limit the extent of the body's natural recovery

---

Classifying an injury

It's important to understand that the physical consequences of a spinal cord injury vary with its location and severity. This dictates which parts of the body and organ systems are affected and influences the expectations (not least in the minds of the medical professionals) for treatment and the potential for recovery, determining what therapy they offer in the phases of treatment.

When your nervous system is working properly, it carries messages to and from your brain and body parts. The nervous system is complex, but in essence, these messages control at least three important functions:

1. The motor functions that determine your ability to control the contraction of your muscles consciously and deliberately, and hence the movement of your limbs to carry out everyday tasks.

2. The sensory functions that reflect the sensation of touch: your ability to 'feel' things and be aware of the position of your limbs in space even with your eyes closed.

3. The autonomic functions, which refer to actions that your brain controls without you having to think about them. Your heart beating and your lungs taking a breath are examples. Interestingly, just because functions are autonomic, it does not mean that you have no ability to consciously influence them. The autonomic nervous system (ANS) has a powerful effect on many organ systems and is central to how we all behave under stress – we will explore this in more detail in Chapter Three.

In basic terms, the closer the damage to the spinal cord is to the head and neck, the more parts of the body are affected and potentially the greater the degree of disability. This is because the nerves at a vertebra represent a part of the communication path between the brain and the various body systems below that level.

When the spinal cord is damaged, messages cannot 'jump over' the damaged area. In other words, the messages sent from the brain cannot make it to body parts below the damaged area, and vice versa. Thus, the body at and below the level of injury is affected, but our bodies are resilient, and the nervous system will attempt to 'rewire' itself and work around the problem. Current research and clinical practice encourage this process, as we will learn later.

As we learned at the start of this chapter, the ASIA system is recognised internationally as the way to classify spinal cord injuries, and it can also classify improvements over time. As you might expect, it is used to group and compare patients and predict functional outcomes for rehabilitation.

The definition of spinal cord injury levels and the classification of the injury can seem confusing if you haven't met them before. A basic description of injury at various levels is:

- **Cervical.** The neck area contains seven cervical vertebrae (C1 to C7) and eight cervical nerves (C1 to C8). Cervical injuries usually cause loss of function in the chest, arms and legs. They can also affect breathing and bowel and bladder control.

These effects are in addition to loss of function in the thoracic, lumbar and sacral regions.

- **Thoracic.** At the central chest area there are twelve thoracic vertebrae (T1 to T12) and twelve thoracic nerves (T1 to T12). Thoracic spinal cord injuries usually affect the chest and the legs. Injuries to the upper thoracic area can affect breathing. Thoracic injuries can also affect bowel and bladder control.

- **Lumbar.** The lumbar area (between the chest and the pelvis) contains five vertebrae (L1 to L5) and five nerves. Lumbar injuries usually affect the hips and legs, and can also affect bowel and bladder control.

- **Sacral.** The sacral area (from the pelvis to the end of the spine) contains five sacral vertebrae (S1 to S5) and five sacral nerves (S1 to S5). Sacral spinal cord injuries usually affect the hips and legs. Injuries to the upper sacral area can also affect bowel and bladder control.

For example, in an injury between C1 and C8, messages to and from the brain are stopped in the neck area. This usually results in at least some paralysis of the chest, arms and legs (tetraplegia, also known as quadriplegia). In an L3 injury, messages are stopped at the lower back. This results in at least some paralysis of the legs and hips, which is referred to as paraplegia.

As we learned earlier, injuries are also described as complete or incomplete. The ASIA system further classifies incomplete injuries into four subsections:

- **A: Complete.** No feeling or movement of the areas of your body that are controlled by your lowest sacral nerves. This means you do not have feeling around the anus or control of the muscle that closes the anus, so people with complete spinal cord injuries do not have control of bowel and bladder function.

- **B: Incomplete.** There is feeling, but no movement below the level of injury, including sacral segments that control bowel and bladder function.

- **C: Incomplete.** There is both some feeling and movement below the level of injury. More than half of the key muscles can move, but not strongly enough to generate movement against gravity. Moving against gravity means, for example, raising your hand to your mouth when you are sitting up.

- **D: Incomplete.** There is both some feeling and movement below the level of injury. More than half of the key muscles can move against gravity.

- **E: Incomplete.** Feeling and movement are normal, though there may be damage to vertebrae.

In summary, an injury is described as complete if there is no voluntary motor (movement) or sensory function below the level of injury. If the arms are spared, the injured person has paraplegia. If they are involved, the person has tetraplegia. The level of injury is the lowest intact spinal cord segment.

Consequences of the level of injury

It is completely rational that in the early phases of treatment, surgical and medical care is tailored to the needs of the individual and based on the specific nature of their injury. Once rehabilitation starts in hospital, the therapy provided will also be tailored to some extent to the level of injury and will aim to teach self-care and everything the injured person needs to maximise independence.

Patients can get frustrated when they perceive fellow patients to be receiving 'more therapy' than they are themselves – you will read some examples in the cases I describe in this book. This is because their assumed potential for recovery to some extent dictates how scarce resource is provided in the hospital system. Once we recognise that regaining some control is a fundamental driver for any person in this situation, this frustration becomes understandable. I have never met anyone who's complained they received too much therapy.

The danger comes when shortage of resource is the real driver for what happens clinically rather than the injured person's potential for benefit. In the past, many rehabilitation programmes have relied mainly on expert opinion, but evidence-based approaches are now becoming more apparent. In addition to the ASIA score, other measures that may be used in clinical practice include the Spinal Cord Independence Measure and Walking Index for Spinal Cord Injury II (WISCI II) scale, and the Short-form Health Survey (SF-36) quality of life test. These useful measurements are intended to aid decision making for treatment and rehabilitation, taking into consideration the individual's capacity and expectation to reintegrate into society.

Limitations of an ASIA score

I have met lots of people who initially see their ASIA classification as an absolute marker of what is going to be possible for them. From the clinical-management point of view, it is essential to have measurement tools, but patients can see these as representing insurmountable barriers. Then they are surprised that a later therapy intervention reveals function they believe they are 'not supposed to have'.

Spinal cord injuries are highly variable. We can only compare two people, both with injuries to their spine and even with the same ASIA score, cautiously with respect to their capabilities or functional recovery patterns. Spinal cord injuries are also highly heterogeneous, which means it is challenging to assess the value of treatments to individuals. An accurate ASIA score is useful – after all, that is its intention – but never consider it a 'tablet of stone'.

An optimistic view of spinal cord injuries is that most are in a practical sense incomplete – even the ones that seem otherwise. This suggests that many patients have an ability to transmit information from the brain to affected muscles through spared, albeit fragmented, neural networks. In addition, when we consider that an injury that damages the spinal cord often spares the brain, the advantage of an incomplete injury becomes even more powerful.

An incomplete injury suggests a great opportunity for functional recovery. It does not make recovery easy, though, and experts are still striving to learn how to take advantage of this potential.

KEY POINT

It is important to find out as much as possible about your specific level of injury and its nature. Many people who are told they have a complete injury believe that this always means their cord is totally cut through or that certain activities are not going to be productive, so they may feel that it's not worth trying in their rehabilitation, but this is not necessarily the case.

It is tough to challenge medical authority. If you are doing so, make sure that your safety comes first, but there is a good reason to learn about your specific injury. Once you know more, you don't have to speculate and risk fuelling fear and uncertainty. Instead, you can take back control and make plans for the future.

Summary

Basic statistics about a condition such as a spinal cord injury, which is potentially so catastrophic, have not in the past been as detailed as we might like. In the UK, the numbers injured each year are around 2,500 with the age profile shifting towards an older demographic with many more incomplete injuries. Resources to help people with this condition are not adequate and many are not even able to access the specialist treatment provided by the spinal-injury units.

The severity of the impact a spinal cord injury has on the person depends on its location and their medical management from the moment of injury. An ASIA score describes much of the character of an injury at a particular point in time and its impact on sensory and motor functions, but it is not an absolute marker of rehabilitation potential. Everyone will exhibit some unique characteristics that complicate any attempts to group people by ASIA score and predict outcomes for rehabilitation.

All spinal cord injuries are medical emergencies and are usually described as having primary and secondary phases. Medical interventions in the early stages of injury are tailored to the events that arise as the body strives to repair itself and aim to prevent the secondary complications that can occur and delay subsequent rehabilitation. Most injuries are incomplete, which implies that there is some capacity for functional recovery providing that appropriate steps are taken. At the time of writing, though, we are still in the early stages of understanding how best to maximise recovery.

The Christopher Reeve story

Those of us of a certain age will remember Christopher Reeve for his leading role in the film *Superman* in 1978, and then as the man who shone a new light on spinal cord injury and its treatment. Reeve's injury in 1995 was at high level on the spinal cord, resulting in quadriplegia; he used a wheelchair and ventilator for the rest of his life. For those of us involved in rehabilitation, he is best remembered for the creation of the Christopher and Dana Reeve Foundation and its ongoing mission of curing spinal cord injury.

Personally, I remember that he was responsible for questioning some of the accepted wisdom about the potential for recovery following an injury. The scientific literature on spinal cord injury at the time predicted that most recovery should occur in the first six months after injury and generally complete within two years. Reeve's partial recovery, coming some five to seven years after his injury, defied these medical expectations and had a dramatic effect on his daily life.

He recovered some movement and sensation that medical science at the time suggested he could never have. He was never able to walk again, he did not regain bowel, bladder or sexual function, but his limited recovery was still considered significant as it defied expectations. What is accepted wisdom at some point in time often proves to be far from wise later.

Reeve himself believed his improved function was the result of intense physical exercise. Five years after his injury, Reeve noticed that he could voluntarily move an index finger, and then he began an intense exercise programme. He used daily electrical muscle stimulation to build mass in his arms and legs, rode an FES cycling system, did spontaneous breathing training and participated in hydrotherapy. In 1998 and 1999, Reeve underwent treadmill training to encourage functional stepping.

This single case does not prove there is a generalised cause-and-effect relationship between exercise and functional recovery, but Reeve's treating physicians certainly believed that his intensive exercise programme was responsible for the benefits he experienced. What is never in doubt is that exercise leads to better health in everyone.

You could argue that Reeve's participation in such intense exercise was possible because he had wealth and fame, but to commit to exercise in the way he did, he still had to overcome the dogma that he should just accept his condition and move on emotionally. He had always been a strong, fit and healthy person prior to his injury, so yes, his participation in exercise was motivated by its well-known benefits on cardiovascular function, muscle tone and bone density, but we can all learn from the positive results he experienced.

After increasing his participation in exercise, Reeve suffered fewer medical complications such as bladder and lung infections. Before 1999, he frequently required hospitalisation – he had a total of nine life-threatening complications and required almost 600 days of antibiotic treatment. From 1999 until his death in 2004, he was not hospitalised at all, had just the one serious medical complication and needed only sixty days of antibiotic treatment. These improvements in his health boosted Reeve's emotional wellbeing and enabled him to commit to a variety of work projects knowing he could give them his uninterrupted attention. He debuted as a film director and starred in an updated version of the classic Hitchcock thriller *Rear Window*, for which he was nominated for a Golden Globe Award and won the Screen Actors Guild Award for Outstanding Performance by a Male Actor in a Television Movie or Miniseries.

Christopher Reeve's case and the foundation created by him and his wife have helped to change experts' thinking and expectations for spinal cord rehabilitation.

TWO
The Evolution Of Treatment

We should never be arrogant about how much we know today because it is almost certain that our knowledge is not as complete as we would like to think. Around 250 years ago, Voltaire is reputed to have said:

> 'Doctors prescribe medicine of which they know little, to cure diseases of which they know less, in human beings of which they know nothing.'

This quote is as relevant today as it was centuries ago, but I don't look upon it as a criticism of medical science. It is a pointer to the complexity of human physiology, and of health and disease. This stuff is difficult, but we are getting better at it. Eric Topol MD, who has become something of an evangelist for change in the medical profession, wrote in his book *The Creative Destruction of Medicine* (Topol, 2012):

> 'Of all the professions represented on the planet, perhaps none is more resistant to change than physicians.'

There is no doubt that doctors, like all of us, need to learn to take advantage of the impact of technology and continually strive to grasp new knowledge in their field. Whatever era we live in, ways of doing things never stay the same for too long, but in clinical medicine, there is the imperative to 'first do no harm' and this means that changes in practice tend to be slow and measured. We strive to be safe as well as effective. Dramatic change will usually only follow dramatic events.

In this chapter, we will look at the tremendous progress that has been made in treating spinal cord injuries. To set goals in life, we must look ahead with ambition, but to measure our progress, we should look back from time to time. If we are always looking forward, progress towards our goals can seem so slow that we can lose heart. By looking back, we can see more clearly just how far we have come, and this gives us fresh energy to act today.

The emergence of specialist care

Injury to the spinal cord has been with us since humans first walked upon the planet, but there was

THE EVOLUTION OF TREATMENT

no practical improvement in treatment and there were certainly no dedicated spinal-injury units until the beginning of the twentieth century. Injury to the spinal cord itself cannot be repaired yet and treatment over the years has largely consisted of preventing complications until the bony spine and body systems stabilised. Once medically stable, the person could then be rehabilitated to the greatest degree of independence deemed possible at the time.

In the early twentieth century up to the start of the First World War in 1914, physiotherapy and rehabilitation were not the recognised specialities we see today. Various forms of trauma treatment were used in the UK at this time, such as massage, limb manipulation, hydrotherapy and the curious 'application of electricity', all of which were to some extent imported from the USA. Dr Silas Weir Mitchell, an outstanding American neurologist, had developed a treatment there in the 1870s based on his experience with casualties in the American Civil War. This regime stressed bed rest, massage, electrotherapy and 'aggressive feeding', which doesn't sound too good, but refers to high protein feeding to counter the catabolic state typical in the weeks following injury. Mitchell relied on the help of a team of nurse-masseuses, whom he believed (Mitchell, 1877):

> '... should be young, refined and cheerful, gentle but firm, intelligent enough to converse with her patient on matters of the day and able to write a good letter.'

Mitchell demanded absolute obedience to his regime and isolated his patients from outside influences. He is said to have had some success in relative terms, but I'm not sure this approach would meet with approval today. Even at the time, this scheme was somewhat controversial, but not because of obvious gender stereotyping. The two most influential British orthopaedic surgeons of the era, Hugh Owen Thomas and Robert Jones, would especially not allow movement or massage and devised splints to immobilise a fractured body part. They believed that it was 'the prerogative of Nature alone' to repair the body and that total rest was needed, which was very much a case of eminence-based rather than evidence-based medicine.

Electrotherapy, as it was applied at the time, was controversial too. Although widely used from the eighteenth century onward, the techniques had become misappropriated by charlatans who undermined the efforts of more serious clinicians and scientists. Nonetheless, an 'electrical machine' was installed in the Middlesex Hospital in London in 1768, and by 1836 Guy's Hospital had created an electrical department with the respected physicist Golding Bird in charge. Electrotherapy in various forms still has (and deserves) a place in modern therapy, although its practice is thankfully more refined today.

We'll now look at the arrival of the first spinal-injury units, which set the tone for contemporary care in recent times. The interested reader can review the history of the treatment of spinal injuries in extensive detail in the book of the same name (Silver, 2003).

The first spinal-injury units

The First World War led to the development of the first identifiable spinal-injury unit as a practical necessity. In the early part of the war, hospitals were becoming crowded with 'incurable' paralysed patients. Following an appeal in the *Times of London* newspaper and a public demand to 'do something', the Red Cross opened the first Royal Star and Garter Home in Richmond with sixty-four beds. Those patients with spinal cord or brain injuries who survived the early consequences of battlefield trauma were transferred to chronic rehabilitation units at Lonsdale House, the Royal Star and Garter Home and Rookwood.

There is no official history of the treatment available at the Royal Star and Garter Home in the early days, but visiting consultants and medical staff described patients who were 'totally disabled and confined to bed, with persistent urinary tract infections, kidney stones and recurrent pressure sores' (Silver, 2003). This contrasts strongly with the reports from residents who optimistically described being mobilised and discharged home.

The Royal Star and Garter Home carried out forms of rehabilitation from the outset – but not rehabilitation as we might envisage it today. Facilities were provided for handicraft, needlework and embroidery, shoe making and repairs, leather, cane and woodwork, along with recreational and sports facilities. Residents also practised salmon fly dressing, painting, watchmaking and repairing.

An important point to make is that at this time, disabled people were generally institutionalised to receive long-term care or left to the mercy of their families or charity. Within the Royal Star and Garter Home, they were supported by the Ministry of Pensions, but no thought was given to supporting patients being discharged into the community.

The professionals at the home recognised the need to get people near to their families but understood the difficulty of providing special equipment at the patient's home or local hospital. In the home's exercise room, patients were mobilised and taught to walk whenever possible with the aid of sticks or crutches. Orthotic bracing with inside irons, T-straps and toe-raising springs were used. Motorised attachments were available for wheelchairs to create assistive technology to compensate for a patient's disabilities.

Sir Ludwig Guttmann

Ludwig Guttmann was the first director of the new Stoke Mandeville Spinal Injuries Unit in 1944. I mention his story here because he is pretty much the initiator of the approaches embedded in practice today.

Guttmann had escaped from Germany with his family in 1939 and initially commenced work as a research fellow at the Nuffield Department of Neurosurgery in Oxford. He was not allowed to treat patients in this first post due to the differences in medical approaches

THE EVOLUTION OF TREATMENT

between Germany and Britain; his qualifications were not accepted as 'suitable', which he must have found frustrating.

Once at Stoke Mandeville, he was at last able to exercise complete control in his role. Because the field of spinal cord injury was not recognised as important or popular by the medical establishment (the results of treatment were still generally considered to be poor), he was not as subject to the approval of others.

Although Guttmann was said to have taken most of his early ideas for application in Stoke Mandeville from Dr Donald Munro, this is probably to his credit rather than something to criticise him for. Munro had created the first effective treatment for spinal injuries at the City Hospital in Boston, USA, taking what we would now call a holistic approach, and is considered by many today to be the father of paraplegia. He was innovative in both the clinical details and the broader aspects of spinal cord injury management, recognising the benefits of physiotherapy and the need for patient's skin to be protected from developing pressure ulcers, describing rhizotomy techniques to eliminate spasms and designing ways to prevent urinary infections.

Guttmann was passionate about clinical research and meticulous in applying his methods. Although his German qualifications were not readily accepted at first, there is no doubt that Guttmann was well trained in several fields including neurology, neurosurgery, research methodology and rehabilitation. Under Guttmann's leadership, Stoke Mandeville gained dynamism because the patient always came first in the German system, which was not always the case in UK teaching hospitals at the time.

By the time of his arrival at Stoke Mandeville, Guttmann had a lot of practical experience in treating peripheral nerve injuries and saw value in using this as the foundation of his treatment of spinal cord injuries. His clinical education in the German system meant that he did not want to be subject to the limited time slots available to examine patients that were typical of a UK teaching hospital of the time. Instead, his methodology involved the presentation of individual cases, tutorials and lectures. He examined every new case that was admitted in detail, and then presented it along with treatment recommendations at weekly teaching sessions that would last into the night.

Guttmann recognised that leadership is an essential ingredient for success and is reported to have been an inspiring man who uplifted the morale of patients and staff alike. He was an innovator in the field and demonstrated that something worthwhile could be done for spinal-injury patients.

Guttmann wrote in the *Medical Times* (Guttmann, 1945):

'Positive proof of recuperation is invaluable in convincing the man that hope is not lost – over-cheerfulness and self-deception, which some of these cases show, also need attention at later stages.'

THE EVOLUTION OF TREATMENT

In his early days at Stoke Mandeville, it sounds like Guttmann upset a few traditional ways of doing things. Undeterred, he used his charisma to make sure his will was carried out. For example, he dictated that all patients be turned every two hours, day and night, whether the patient was sleeping or not. Staff who were expected to follow these orders were not happy, so he made surprise visits to wards at all hours to make sure that they were kept on their toes. This approach helped prevent ulcers that resulted from unremitting pressure on insensitive paralysed tissue.

In his private moments, Guttmann said that other people had developed aspects of his treatment, but his own achievement was to bring all these ideas together in an integrated programme. In 1955, Reginald Watson-Jones, an eminent figure in UK orthopaedics, commented on the remarkable work being carried out by Guttmann at Stoke Mandeville (Watson-Jones, 1955):

> 'Not only has he cured neglected decubitus ulcers, contractures of joints and spasms of the lower limbs in patients with traumatic paraplegia of long standing, but above all, he has inspired them with a new faith and new hope.'

Faith and hope are powerful forces that we should always encourage when they stem from effective action and know-how. Faith and hope without action are hollow and meaningless. If life feels like it is out of control for someone, it becomes easy for them to default to a state of hopelessness.

KEY POINT

Specialist treatment units were created based on methods originating in the USA and refined by Ludwig Guttmann at Stoke Mandeville in the late 1940s. These efforts changed the world view of spinal cord injury to the much more positive perspective that we see today, which means it's not a massive effort now to train hopefulness into our healthcare systems.

The democratisation of healthcare

When I show new rehabilitation technology to healthcare professionals, they rightly ask, 'Where is the evidence that shows the value of this?' However, not all healthcare professionals understand how to gain evidence of effectiveness or the limitations of the standard research approaches (which were often developed to be used with medications) when it comes to looking at rehabilitation and related technology. Developing a totally evidence-based health service, vital though it may seem to be, is a complex undertaking. If we get it wrong, we may stifle innovation along with our desire to prevent harm.

Medical care today is largely shaped by guidelines for clinical effectiveness which are indexed to a large statistical population rather than the needs of an individual. The holy grail of evidence-based medicine has been the randomised large-scale double-blind placebo-controlled trial. This means that typically, 10,000

THE EVOLUTION OF TREATMENT

or more patients are randomly assigned to take a drug or a placebo (more about this in a moment) without the patient or their doctor knowing what they received.

On the face of it, this approach seems to make sense. The logic that applies is if an intervention works for many people with few side effects, this must be a good thing. The truth is that this approach does not easily translate to the real-world needs of the individual person for rehabilitation. This does not even work well for drug trials anymore because there is often a large amount of individual variation in how patients respond to any drug. Large differences also exist between male and female responses to many drugs.

We have seen great advances in medical care that have consigned many infectious diseases that once shortened lives to being a thing of the past. Critical care and trauma management have also improved dramatically in recent decades. Chronic conditions and physical rehabilitation provide a different and difficult challenge because there is a greater need for individualised care and our present systems of care delivery are not optimised for this.

People who have had a spinal cord or any catastrophic injury are not one homogenous population all carrying the same functional disabilities. Consequently, it's difficult or even impossible to use research approaches that were originally devised to study the effects of medication with large populations for personalised rehabilitation. Once a person in the UK with a spinal cord injury has moved beyond the initial stage of treatment and is medically stable, they may find that what the NHS can offer is not going to be sufficient to exploit their full potential for recovery. They may even have been labelled as having 'no further potential for improvement' to formally end an episode of care for administrative reasons.

In rehabilitation, the care pathways for spinal cord injury are robust and effective for dealing with the acute stage of managing the injured person, but once they are medically stable, they need a much more individualised approach. Someone needs to assess the individual's potential for progress, identify some realistic goals, marshal resources and get to work.

Contrast this with a trend – described by Eric Topol (2012) as mass medicalisation – in healthcare towards prescribing medications as primary prevention, for example, the drive to prescribe statins to men over fifty years of age. These trends, acting on the population statistics of evidenced-based medicine, have been criticised in some quarters because for an individual, statistics can be misleading. If a statin reduces the risk of having a heart attack by 36%, this sounds like great news until we recognise that around 3% of patients taking a placebo had a heart attack compared with 2% taking a particular statin. In other words, for every 100 patients taking a statin, only one was helped and ninety-nine were not. With mass medicalisation we are increasing the cost of healthcare with little certainty of benefit for any individual; in fact, the individual is much more likely to suffer side effects of the medication than be helped (Topol, 2012).

At present, we have limited insight into the physiology of each individual. Understandably, the life-science industry is not motivated to design drugs or medical devices that are only effective for a small well-defined segment of the population. Increasing costs, low patent lives and diminishing returns from the traditional drug development processes have also led to a complete rethink about the future of life science. At the same time, the regulatory authorities are risk averse and sometimes suppress innovative or even the most frugal opportunities to change medicine.

At the present time, the medical device regulations around the world are changing dramatically, leading to many smaller companies deciding they cannot continue to offer medical technology. Safety must come first, but by acting as if everything must be tested like a drug, we may have stifled innovation for a generation.

KEY POINT

Rehabilitation is perhaps not the sexiest branch of medicine, but it is extremely challenging and vital for optimal recovery. An individualised approach is needed once the person is medically stable, informed but not constrained by their ASIA score.

In the UK, individualised therapy is going to be challenging for the NHS to deliver to everyone with the resources available, so I'm encouraging you to learn as much as possible about your condition and potential for recovery as the springboard to help yourself.

Summary

The treatment of spinal cord injuries has progressed dramatically in the last 100 years, although a total cure has remained elusive. Systems of care have been developed to improve the prospects for rehabilitation, but much remains to be done. Medical science will probably always be reluctant to change as any new intervention has to be not only safe, but effective, which can be hard to pin down.

The first UK spinal-injury units were formed as a response to battlefield trauma and evolved to improve survival and standards of care. With improved treatments, patients were offered rehabilitation at first in institutions and latterly at home. Sir Ludwig Guttmann, among others, raised the standards of care as well as the expectations of survivors. He brought both quality and quantity of life to survivors; he also brought hope.

In the UK, injured people today have high expectations of the NHS, but it is difficult for individualised and intensive rehabilitation to be offered by a system that is attuned to providing healthcare to a general population with disparate needs and wants.

Mark Pollock's story

In 1998, Mark Pollock was a student at Trinity College, Dublin, looking forward to his final exams in Business Studies and Economics when he suddenly lost his sight. Over the next ten years, he rebuilt his life and exceeded his pre-blindness achievements.

In 2002, the former Irish international rower won bronze and silver medals for Northern Ireland in the Commonwealth Rowing Championships. In 2003, he ran six marathons in seven days across the Gobi Desert. In 2004, he completed the North Pole Arctic Marathon. In 2009, Mark became the first blind man to reach the South Pole. Using insights from these and many other extreme challenges, he launched a successful leadership and motivational speaking business to inspire people in companies to adapt, perform and collaborate to achieve more.

In 2010, Mark's life took a turn once again when he fell from a second storey window and experienced a spinal cord injury at T9 and L1. I met Mark and his fiancée, Simone, in Stoke Mandeville's Spinal Unit in October 2010 when I was introduced to him by another patient. Mark persuaded me to test his leg muscles to see if they would contract with electrical stimulation.

It was quite likely that his level of spinal cord injury would result in what is called muscle denervation. If muscles are denervated, they will change their structure over time. In a few years, the size and quality of the muscle tissue will have gone and been replaced by fat and connective tissue. I would not have expected his leg muscles to respond to conventional electrical stimulation as this relies on the local nerve supply being intact and his injury was likely to have disrupted the so-called lower motor neurons responsible for this.

Sure enough, on testing, I found weak muscle contractions occurred on his left quadriceps, left calf and pre-tibial muscles. The right quadriceps only showed a light flicker of a contraction deep in the leg.

According to my notes at the time, Mark stated, 'I have no feeling or movement from my belly button down. However, the left side feeling goes slightly below the belly button. Plus, my abs are contracting, albeit weakly, far below my belly button.'

Conventional wisdom at the time said that Mark would be unlikely to benefit from electrical stimulation or FES cycling since the denervation injury would mean that his muscles would not respond and contract in a useful way. This was the opinion of the therapists at the spinal unit, and it was also my opinion. What happened next rewrote my beliefs about what to expect.

Mark is a determined and persistent individual. If he has a goal or a belief, he will pursue it relentlessly, despite the apparent obstacles in the way. He wasn't allowed to use electrical stimulation in the spinal unit, but he 'arm twisted' me to use FES as soon as he had left hospital. We created a series of programmes to stimulate his leg muscles in sequence, even though I told him this wasn't likely to be productive.

After three months, I got a phone call from Mark to tell me that he was now able to get clear muscle contractions in both legs. This implied some recovery of the nervous system structure within the leg muscles; something that I had not expected. This led to us working much more deliberately to restore denervated muscle via specifically tailored electrotherapy, which we will look at later in this book.

At the time I first met him, Mark had created a great career as a leadership and motivational speaker based on his ability to move beyond the challenges of blindness and set goals, put teams together and take on endurance challenges in harsh environments. After his spinal injury, he was honest enough to say that he didn't have a clue how he would manage with two disabilities. How could he get in front of an audience of businesspeople and talk about motivation and overcoming life's obstacles if he wasn't able to demonstrate this himself?

Step forward a few years and Mark's career is very much back on track and making an impact – this time on a global scale. He continues to pioneer the use of therapeutic interventions in partnership with scientists and technologists, and he is working to bring people together to cure paralysis in our lifetime. If you are curious about what Mark has achieved and what he is doing now, check out his site at www.markpollock.com. He has lots of content, TED talks and a full-length movie *Unbreakable* that is worth watching.

Mark is a person who pushes the boundaries of what his body is capable of and challenges conventional thinking about the correct course of action. I told him that his muscles would not respond to electrical stimulation as that was the prevailing view. It turned out that Mark was right to challenge me just as he challenges himself every day.

THREE
Assorted Mind Games

A spinal cord injury initiates a difficult journey no one ever wants to take. If this has happened to you, I'm sure you can think of other metaphors to describe what it is like. In the early stages of recovery, medical science dictates what happens and usually there is not much you can, or should, do about that. At some point, though, you will be medically stable and can think about your own goals for the future and your version of recovery. Although you are likely to be influenced by others, this is the stage of the journey where you start to have some control over what happens.

There isn't much in the way of maths in this book, but let's try out a little equation inspired by one of my favourite business coaches, Timothy Gallwey (2000):

Your performance = Your potential
minus interference

What you can achieve in any situation is hardly ever equal to your potential. There are always sources of interference and the most significant tends to be you yourself. A little self-doubt and some erroneous assumptions, often triggered by bad advice from well-meaning people, coupled with fear of failure can sabotage progress.

Being realistic

Our mindset, attitudes and beliefs are often not in our conscious awareness, but in all walks of life, they are potentially powerful sources of interference. Conversely, they can be positive resources that help us reach our goals.

When you read the stories in this book, notice how much each person's mindset affected their results. You may be tempted to think that these people are naturally tough and resilient – it looks that way on the surface, but don't mistake external signs of toughness for inner confidence and drive. Just like you and me, they will have struggled with self-doubt and feelings of powerlessness, but they learned to be resourceful.

When we peek below the surface, we are initially all the same when faced with a catastrophic injury. When control and choice seem to be taken away from us, we go into what is called 'learned helplessness' – in other words, we do not act and cannot think clearly.

We lose sight of our future path. It's then that we need hope, but it must be realistic.

For some of my clients, imagining the future in six months, a year or even ten years helps them move on from helplessness. This is not some wild fantasy; they appreciate the things that will still be there, such as the love of a partner, the beauty of the changing seasons, the affection of family and so on. These significant things that it's so easy to take for granted remind them that whatever they are going through is temporary.

Other clients seek something they can act on. They learn as much as they can about their situation, then armed with that knowledge, they take action – however small – to move them forward. True confidence for them comes from making an effort, which brings the sense of control that's so essential for all humans. They see progress, even if their overarching goal is not yet within reach.

You can learn to be realistic about your hopes and goals by balancing two things:

- An accurate appraisal of your condition and its demands
- An accurate assessment of your ability to change things for the better

A clinician who encourages you to be 'realistic' about your prospects for recovery always means well, but if they make this comment thoughtlessly, they may stifle hope just when you need it most. At the other extreme, forget audacious goals that will only set you up for failure. Somewhere in the middle lies your individual potential for recovery.

For example, it doesn't matter how hard I believe and dream about it, I will never be the heavyweight boxing champion of the world. There are always limits, but if I make the effort, I can become a better boxer within the constraints of my physique.

It is often useful to become knowledgeable about your condition, then aware of your own attitudes and beliefs. Notice how they are affecting your feelings and behaviour, and choose to adopt those that will serve you best. How can you respond resourcefully rather than reactively?

Most people allow their ideas about what is possible to be shaped by what they think is their reality. In fact, for all of us, 'reality' is built from our ideas and patterns of belief. It's not always easy to choose supportive attitudes and beliefs, but it's a skill worth learning. The real toughness you need when experiencing distress is about paying attention to your feelings, leaning in and creating mental space to take thoughtful action.

KEY POINT

Whenever we face a massive challenge, we have expectation and we have reality. When these are far apart, we have a problem. We need expectation and reality to overlap.

A better you

Young children have an amazing ability to switch between emotions. One moment, they laugh with joy, then they cry. Another moment, and they're dancing and singing. They have an emotional flexibility that most of us lose as we get older and the deep and often negative patterns of our attitudes and beliefs – patterns we likely don't even know we have – become ruts.

Have you noticed that when people say they feel bad and you ask them why, they tend to start their reply with the word 'because'? This points to their belief that something outside of themselves or their control is the cause of their bad feelings. As many of the biggest upsets and dramatic changes in life are outside of our control, most of us are at the mercy of 'be-cause'.

Young children are masters at generating strong emotions, but they are not so good at regulating them. That's the skill we need to discover as adults facing a challenge. Psychology is still looking for the 'silver bullet' to manage our emotions. Coping or avoidance strategies that work for one person don't necessarily work for another, so we need the flexibility to use different strategies and the capacity to be able to draw upon them. The intensity of the situation matters, too.

In her second book, *The Bigger Picture*, written following her spinal cord injury, Claire Lomas (2022) notes: 'Before my accident I had clear directions in life, then it was like the 5,000-piece jigsaw shattered.' We all need to know how to put the pieces back together.

Throughout history, humans have sought personal meaning and purpose in their lives. In his book *The Hero with a Thousand Faces*, author Joseph Campbell (1949) pointed to how each life can be seen as a journey: a hero's journey with definite stages identified in a so-called Monomyth that crosses the world's cultures. It was also Joseph Campbell who pointed to the fact that life is a bit like going to the cinema and finding the movie is already playing. You have to watch for quite a while before you get a feel for the plot, then just as you start to get comfortable with what is going on, someone taps you on the shoulder and tells you it's time to leave.

None of us can control all aspects of life and it can be painful to have a reminder of this when fate strikes. It's helpful to remember that we do all have a purpose and can find meaning in life – not some great scheme, but the small acts that bring joy to ourselves and others.

Claire Lomas, who we will learn more about at the end of this chapter, found purpose by sharing her story and raising funds to support research. Mark Pollok challenged his own body to discover the frontiers of what is possible following a spinal cord injury while inspiring others around the world to join the cause to find a cure. In both cases, these people's drivers for purpose didn't emerge fully formed, but came about through small actions they took over a period.

It is obvious that a spinal cord injury will result in emotional as well as physical trauma, so to get life back on track, we need to deal with both in one way or another. Feeling bad for too long causes stress, ages our bodies, adds to our burden of sickness and leaves us powerless to shape our present and future – we will explore why this is so in a moment.

I can't emphasise enough the importance of this. It's the difference between being swept along by 'be-cause' and regaining control. High performers, whether in sport or business, learn to access resourceful states at will and there are several ways (both ancient and modern) to do this, as we will discover later in the chapter. It's not necessarily the intellectual act of 'thinking', but self-awareness that is the first step to being resourceful.

Some understanding of how our mind-body system works can help point the way, so let's take a closer look at aspects of our physiology. For a long time, neuroscientists agreed that emotions are shaped by certain parts of the brain. More recently, we have discovered that this view of the brain as the 'master organ' is an oversimplification. In fact, the brain and the body have a huge collective impact on our emotions. It's a two-way street. Our feelings and how we use or move our bodies can change our brain just as our brain can change our feelings and the state of our body systems.

As long ago as 1884, American psychologist William James (1948) published an essay entitled 'What is an emotion?' based on his observations as a philosopher and his knowledge of physiology. He believed that the source of emotions is purely visceral, not cognitive – in other words, emotions originate in the organs of the body and not the mind. The idea here is that we perceive events via the senses and as a result have bodily feelings – after the perception, which triggers our memories and imagination, we have a physical sensation that we label as emotion.

James believed that ultimately, there was no such thing as emotion; there was simply perception and a triggered bodily response. The physical sensations that would arise, such as the pounding heart, sweating, tightness in the stomach, tense muscles, were what we call emotions.

James's theories were largely discounted because they were not supported by evidence. In fact, his own student, Walter Cannon had by 1927 explained the workings of what we now know as the sympathetic part of the ANS (Quick et al, 1994). This is the part activated when we are under stress – the so-called fight-or-flight mechanism.

A single nerve, the vagus (which means 'wandering'), exits the back of the brain, then runs down the bundles of nerve cells (ganglia) on either side of the spinal cord. This important nerve sends branches to many body organs including the heart, the pupils of the eye, the salivary glands, the bronchi of the lungs, the adrenal glands and the sex organs. Walter Cannon found that when he stimulated the vagus nerve through electrodes implanted in the hypothalamus area of the brain, he could see rapid physiological changes in all of these organs consistent with how the body would need to respond in emergency situations. From Cannon's point of view, his former teacher's theory of the viscera as the source of emotion was simply not plausible. Cannon saw the hypothalamus as the seat of emotions, which cascaded down to the body through its many neuronal connections.

Nowadays, we have growing scientific evidence that emotions can transform the body – either creating disease or healing it, maintaining health or undermining it. The current 'truth' is that emotions are a property of both the brain and the body. This is a useful paradigm to know.

KEY POINT

Your personal state (that package of your thoughts, feelings, and emotions) absolutely determines what behaviours are possible for you. In other words, if you can find a more resourceful state of mind appropriate to your situation, you can then access better behaviours to deliver better results in your life.

Three principles

There are three principles at work in finding realistic goals appropriate to your situation – awareness, choice and trust, and they are connected. Awareness is about knowing your starting point with absolute clarity and no self-delusion. How can you be realistic about the future if you don't understand where you are starting from? Choice is about moving towards your personal goals with full awareness of the situation. You can be realistic because you have self-awareness, which helps you choose goals that reflect your true self – not those imposed by someone else. Trust is the magic ingredient – a recognition of your inner resources that allows movement towards your goals to take place.

Timothy Gallwey (2000) sees these principles as a cycle with each building on and supporting the others. The more you trust yourself, the easier it is to build awareness. The more aware you are, the greater your choices.

Working in rehabilitation, I find it natural to view the body and its performance in health or disorders as a connected whole. When we actively feel something as an emotion, it is truly engaging our whole physiology, not just our imagination. Although many people remember René Descartes' famous statement, 'I think, therefore I am', a better biological truth would be, 'I *feel*, therefore I am'.

In the distant past, clinicians discovered the physical nerve structure and deduced that this is like the wiring of a telephone exchange, allowing messages to flow back and forth between the brain and the limbs and organ systems. This implied that the nervous system is electrical, but there are in fact at least three types of information flows around our body – physical, electrical and chemical. It's likely you have heard about the electrical information flows along the nerves, such as those that power our muscles or make the sensation of touch possible, as we humans have known about these for longer than the others, which may have come as a surprise.

Science now tells us that every single cell in our body is influenced by our feelings through one aspect of our nervous system and the flow of 'molecules of emotion'. Candace Pert (1997) came up with this term to describe the hormones within our body that act as a type of chemical nervous system, having the power to keep us well or make us ill. These hormones flow through our bloodstream and lymphatic system and can moderate the electrical signals that the nerves are sending.

When electrical messages flow along fibres of the nervous system, the effects are rapid and targeted. Our chemical nervous system acts more slowly than the electrical one and is less specifically targeted, but it's no less important. Hundreds of hormones flow because of our emotions and we manifest the consequence of those feelings. Sad feelings produce sad bodies. Depressed feelings produce depressed and ageing bodies, and happy feelings produce healthy and youthful bodies.

This is important because it implies what science confirms: our feelings and emotions are a factor in the development of cancers, heart attacks and many other damaging events. When people talk about the undesirable aspects of stress, this is, in essence, what they mean.

The physical form of whole-body communication is often forgotten, but is important too (Claxton, 2015).

Whole-body movements carry information and help to coordinate activities going on in different parts of the body. Some effects are apparent to most of us, for example, standing and walking after a large meal aids digestion, and coughing, sneezing and yawning produce pressure waves within the body that pump cerebrospinal fluid to the brain and increase blood flow, but the effects of physical movement can also be subtle. Within the brain, neurons physically twitch and turn when they are activated, and their axons propagate small pressure waves as well as electrical and chemical ones. Even this small-scale physical activity may affect the way messages are routed in the brain, and the way neurons learn.

You might be relieved to know that it is not necessary to understand in detail how the mind-body system works. There are lots of effective mind-body 'hacks', some of which have been around for a thousand years, and later we will look at a few approaches I have experience with. What matters is that you become aware of the importance of your mindset and how this will impact on the way you behave and the results you achieve. For some people, choosing to have a greater self-awareness of and trust in their mindset can be the key to positive change.

KEY POINT

Choose to become aware of the importance of your mindset, and trust in how this will impact on the way you behave and the results you achieve.

The power of the heart

If your partner looked into your eyes and said, 'I love you with all my brain', it wouldn't have quite the same ring of authenticity to it as if they said, 'I love you with all my heart'. For centuries, the heart has been considered the source of emotion, courage and even wisdom, but science is only just getting to grips with the complexity of its influence and what we might do with the knowledge.

Ancient civilisations saw the intellect and emotion, or 'thinking' and 'feeling', as quite separate and often antagonistic functions. In more recent times, many of us, particularly boys, were brought up to have a stiff upper lip and believe that to show any emotion was weakness. No wonder we got used to feeling bad.

We now realise the damage that society does by conditioning people to be 'tough'. In sports, the military and even schools, the belief that people need to be toughened up to produce their best in fact seems to be the cause of poor results and damaged people. It's normal to feel fear when we are in pressure situations. It doesn't mean that we are weak; it's our mind and body trying to protect us. It's literally how we are wired.

The link between the heart and emotion was known and embedded in language and culture long before science had any explanation for this. Although there is still much to learn, we now recognise that high performers in athletics, business, the arts – in fact, high performers of all kinds – often use techniques and approaches such as meditation, biofeedback, neurofeedback or neurolinguistic programming (NLP) to help manage the link between their emotions and performance. These concepts can allow us all to develop a greater personal awareness and an ability to positively influence how we respond to situations that generate strong emotions, whether it's the stress of a real-time situation or anticipation that knocks us off balance.

The ANS

The ANS has two aspects: the sympathetic and parasympathetic. The sympathetic nervous system is powered up in response to our perceiving a stressful event. If only momentarily, we are literally disconnected from the ability to think clearly.

Our physiology was designed for a much simpler life than we face today. Most of us do not have to run from a sabre-toothed tiger demanding we fight or flee. Our stressors in modern society are often subtle – the bill we cannot pay; the aggressive or difficult boss; the person who cuts us up in traffic.

Richard Bandler, the co-founder of NLP, states that our emotions and feelings will affect the quality of our decisions and that better emotions will lead to better decisions (Bandler, 1993). Sounds useful to me, but how do we get ourselves into these emotional states? We can either learn to recognise and then 'manhandle' our emotions into the desired state (challenging for many of us who feel powerless to do this when

ASSORTED MIND GAMES

situations often shape how we feel) or use body and mind together to find better balance using the power intrinsic in the way the heart works.

Far from being a simple pump, the heart both communicates with and influences the brain via the nervous system and the vagus nerve, hormonal system and other pathways. The heart literally acts as if it has a mind of its own. It indirectly affects our creativity, mental clarity, emotional balance and effectiveness.

How does this happen? We humans have long known that changes in our emotions are accompanied by changes in heart rate, blood pressure, respiration, digestion and more. There is a part of our ANS (the sympathetic part) that is mobilised when we are aroused – we are directly energised to fight or flee. In our calmer moments, once the stress situation is gone, another part of our nervous system (the parasympathetic part) damps everything down until our ANS is in balance.

Just breathe

Years ago, as a beginner in a Shotokan karate dojo, I learned how effective breathing can be at keeping me calm. As anyone who has trained in boxing or martial arts will know, sparring can be exhausting for beginners. After a minute, you are gasping for breath due to a mixture of fear and effort. Your heart rate soars and your muscles tend to tense up.

The sensei (instructor) would constantly be barking orders such as 'Control your breath' and 'Slow your breathing; don't gasp'. As my skills developed, I learned how useful breath control was to being effective under pressure. I didn't know about the science then, but learned that how I breathed was one of the easiest ways to find emotional balance. In effect, I was using breath to influence my ANS.

A reasonable assumption would be that the brain is in control of the sympathetic and parasympathetic parts of the ANS, but this only partially matches the true behaviour of our physiology. In fact, there is a neural pathway, so input from the heart to the brain can either inhibit or facilitate the brain's electrical activity via the vagus nerve.

In the 1960s and 1970s, early psychophysiological researchers observed that the heart and brain communicate in ways that significantly affect how we perceive and react to events. The discipline of neurocardiology is still exploring the 'nervous system within the heart' and to some extent, the relationship between emotions and their effect on the destabilisation of the heart continues to be a mystery, but this doesn't mean we can't take advantage of what we do know right now.

The heart's brain

In 1991, Dr JA Armour described the concept of a functional 'heart brain' (Armour, 1991). In his article, he gives an overview of the heart's intrinsic nervous system and the role of both the central and peripheral autonomic neurons in the regulation of cardiac function.

In Dr Armour's model, hormonal, chemical, heart rate and pressure information is translated into neurological impulses and sent from the heart to the brain through several afferent pathways ('afferent' means flowing towards the brain). It is via these nerve pathways that pain signals and other 'feeling' sensations are also sent to the brain.

The afferent nerve pathways enter the brain in the medulla and the signals they carry have a regulatory role over many of the ANS signals that flow from the brain to the heart, blood vessels and other organs and glands. These signals also influence the higher centres of the brain.

Another part of the heart-brain communication system (which is slower acting than the signals carried by the afferent nerve pathways) relates to hormones that are produced and released by the heart. Although science's understanding of this is not perfect, the bottom line is that the heart has its own intrinsic nervous system that can operate and process information independently from the brain.

KEY POINT

We can use body and mind together to find better balance using the power intrinsic in the way the heart works. How we breathe is one of the easiest ways to find emotional balance, in effect using breath to influence our ANS.

Techniques for resourcefulness

Successful people have the ability to trip into a highly resourceful state. Sometimes that state might be relaxed and calm, other times high adrenaline; it depends on the situation. There are lots of ways to do this and we will cover a few in this section. Some techniques are as old as the hills, some more modern, but in my experience, they can all be effective.

Heart focus or centring

The Institute of HeartMath in the USA describes a technique which puts our attention to the heart (Paddison, 1998). This technique, which relies on scientific knowledge about our physiology as well as ancient wisdom, uses the natural power within each of us to achieve ANS balance and reset the amygdala and emotional memory switch. It is a technique that martial artists have known for centuries.

The amygdala is part of the brain which is basically a pattern matching system, constantly looking to identify threats by comparing what is happening at present with our experience. If it perceives a threat, it disconnects us from the cortex and our ability to think clearly and sends a signal via the vagus nerve to the heart that powers us up for fight or flight.

Here is the version of the technique I use within my business. The idea is to catch the stress as soon as the effects surface and transform the negative thoughts

ASSORTED MIND GAMES

and feelings into a positive script leading to action. It takes just a minute to try it.

The key first step is to identify the real nature of the challenge facing you now. This is often difficult as it takes self-awareness to 'catch' your stressed state and choose to take some time out from it, but with practice, this can become automatic for you.

Put your attention to the centre of your chest and breathe in and out smoothly through either the mouth or nose. Don't force your breathing; just let it flow like a tide in and out of the centre of the chest area. If you have difficulty with the concept of putting your attention to your chest, then place a hand there and this will help. Continue to breathe in this way for ten seconds or so.

With your attention on your chest, choose to feel the emotion of love. It could be love you have for a person, a situation, a cherished memory, a pet or even your idea of a perfect day. Recall that emotion and really feel what it was like. It is not important that you see a clear picture; work on the emotion as it is the feeling that matters. If you aren't comfortable with the notion of love, or struggle to think of a situation to experience, activate the feelings of appreciation you have for a place, a person or a thing.

Now ask your heart to give you information about your current challenge that will be of value for you. Trust that it will respond. Both trust and intention are important here; if you doubt this process, you will sabotage your efforts. Listen for the response. It may come in a variety of ways – sometimes immediately and sometimes later.

The abdomen or solar plexus is the centre of balance and the seat of power in martial arts. Anchoring the insights of the heart in this way gives you the strength and commitment to follow through and act on them. This simple technique has a powerful effect in bringing about balance because taking control of your breath and activating strong positive feelings moves your heart rate's variability from chaos to a smoothly changing pattern. This sends a signal to your brain which allows you to find emotional balance once more and think clearly. Sounds like magic, but it is very effective.

The whole body speaks

On a trip to New Zealand, I found a way to get into a highly resourceful state that appeals to my love of martial arts. It is a technique that might well appeal to you too.

Picture the scene. It's a cold and snowy winter morning and I am among a group of visitors at the gates of a prison near Wellington (it's a long story). As the prison gates open, a tattooed warrior appears. With spring-like steps, he moves rapidly towards us with his *taiaha* (a long-handled Māori weapon) at the ready. With wild-eyes and elaborate gestures, he draws a line in the snow on which he places a single fern leaf for us, the visitors. As the warrior withdraws from the line, our leader advances to lift the leaf.

ASSORTED MIND GAMES

For most people, the closest they get to the Māori traditions is watching the *haka* performed by the All Blacks rugby team. The Māori *haka* is normally regarded as a war dance, yet each *haka* has a number of deeper meanings.

Ha means breath; *ka* means to ignite, to energise; so *haka* means to ignite the breath. A great Māori *haka* expert Henare Teowai of the Ngati Porou tribe said that 'the whole body speaks' when it's performed. It is intended to energise the body and inspire the spirit, which sounds to me like getting into a resourceful state.

You can create your own *haka* – a secret personal ritual that ignites your energy and resolve. No one need ever know! What thoughts and memories can you recall right now that put you in a powerful state of mind and body? Remember a time when you felt really inspired. What were you saying? What did you see? What did you hear? How were you standing?

Adopt these same actions if you can, or at least see them in your mind's eye, which is almost as good. Feel the energy flow through you once more. Notice the feelings that swirl around your body and seem to grow stronger. Put these feelings and memories into your own *haka* sequence. It may only be a couple of movements with one or two key words; it doesn't matter – it will work. The intensity and passion are more important than the complexity.

Use this ritual to ignite your breath and power up your energy against your own worst enemy: yourself. Psych yourself up to be your very best every day. If you don't find this easy, you will find some guidance in the bonus content at the end of the book.

Before you dismiss this idea as a bit strange, think about a domain such as sport. Have you noticed how many elite athletes use rituals as part of their performance? At the bottom of all this is the fact that rituals give us a feeling of control and certainty. They are a coping mechanism for the brain and body, convincing us that we have more control than we do.

The Stoic

Stoicism is an ancient philosophy of action that has become popular again. It is embraced by many Silicon Valley entrepreneurs who see it as a practical way of dealing with the inevitable stresses and challenges of their hectic lives. I encourage you to look at it as it might just be something for you. After all, it has survived and thrived for a couple of thousand years.

Stoicism aims to teach us to live by a set of values that contribute to emotional resilience, calm self-confidence and finding a clear direction in life. You could look on it as a guide to life based on reason rather than blind faith that supports you in pursuit of self-mastery, perseverance and wisdom.

The word 'stoicism' has its roots in *stoa*, which is the ancient Greek name for what today we would call a porch, where the Stoics would hang out and talk about enlightenment and 'meaning of life' type stuff. The Greek scholar Zeno is the founder and the

ASSORTED MIND GAMES

Roman emperor Marcus Aurelius the most famous practitioner, while the Roman statesman Seneca is probably the most eloquent and entertaining Stoic, but the real hero of Stoicism, most Stoics agree, is the Greek philosopher Epictetus. He had been a slave, which naturally meant that he would have been familiar with hardship and was probably worth listening to.

Epictetus indirectly taught a whole cast of distinguished people in all walks of life. One of these was the late US Navy Admiral, James Stockdale. A prisoner of war in Vietnam for seven years after being shot down during that conflict, he endured broken bones, starvation, solitary confinement and all manner of torture leading to lifelong disability. His guide and companion through it all were the teachings of Epictetus, with which he had familiarised himself after joining the Navy. He kept those teachings in mind even when things were at their worst.

Stockdale gave a speech at King's College, London in November 1993, which is published as *Courage Under Fire* (Stockdale, 1993). It is well worth a read. He did not buy into the false optimism and wishful thinking of some of his fellow inmates as he saw that was the route to insanity. Through Epictetus, Stockdale found a way to convert adversity into an opportunity.

It boiled down to Stockdale realising that anything outside of the sphere of choice should be considered an opportunity to strengthen our resolve, not an excuse to weaken it. I know that sounds like a challenge, but that to some extent is the point. Only by living through and facing up to adversity can we learn if there is substance to this philosophy.

William B Irvine (2009) suggested that negative visualisation could keep us free from the dangers of too much positive thinking. By keeping the worst that could happen in our heads, we can inoculate ourselves against despair. Only by facing the worst can we come to appreciate the good in the present situation, and then feel gratitude. Gratitude for anything doesn't come easily when we take it for granted.

These principles are suggestive of cognitive behavioural therapy (CBT). Apparently, one of the early developers of CBT read the Stoic philosophers in his youth and was guided by Epictetus's maxim that people are disturbed not by things, but their view of things.

In his *Little Book of Stoicism*, Jonas Salzgeber illustrates the philosophy as the Stoic Happiness Triangle (Salzgeber, 2019). At the centre is the mysterious term 'eudaimonia', which basically means that our purpose is to thrive in our lives; to be supremely happy and in flow.

To live as our best self is not easy, but Stoicism encourages us to do just that. We need to close the gap between what we can do and what we are actually doing. What supports us in this is to focus on what we can control, which is perhaps the most obvious facet of Stoicism. Most of us can get hung up on things we can't control, so this is not easy, but we must accept what already 'is' to be able to flourish.

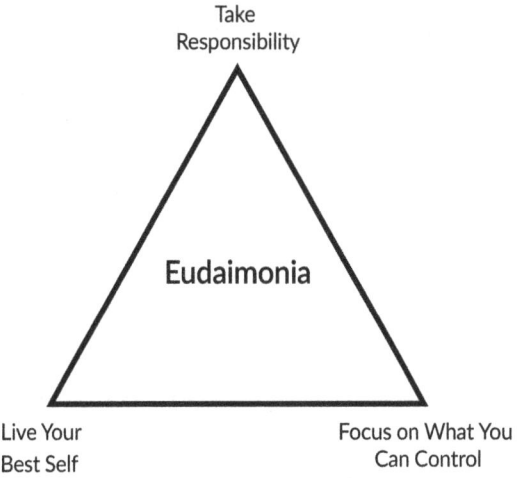

Stoic Happiness Triangle

At the top of the Stoic Happiness Triangle is 'taking responsibility'. The base of the triangle reminds us that external things don't matter when it comes to living a good life. Ultimately, we are responsible because every external thing we can't control offers something that we can control – how we choose to respond to the event.

KEY POINT

Even when events seem beyond your control, you always have control over how you respond to those influences.

Attitudes and beliefs

Let's now talk about attitudes and beliefs, which can be some of the main barriers that pop up whenever we want to set a goal. Goals are obviously important but, as Keith Cunningham (2017) said: 'When it comes to goals, far too much emphasis is placed on visualising Oz and not enough on designing and constructing the yellow brick road.'

This alludes to the difference between actionable plans that lead to meaningful goals and wishful thinking. I meet many people who, following a spinal cord injury, report that their doctors killed their hope. I'm certain that was never the intent, but it is clearly a challenge if those people are to set meaningful goals.

As we learned earlier, Ludwig Guttmann wrote in the *Medical Times* (Guttmann, 1945) that 'Positive proof of recuperation is invaluable in convincing the man that hope is not lost – over-cheerfulness and self-deception, which some of these cases show, also need attention at later stages.'

This suggests finding the balance where hope is tinged with realism. Goals are not plans, merely ideas about possibility, so they could just be wishful thinking. Of course, goals to recover function following a spinal cord injury are emotionally charged and this brings a particular difficulty.

We can never achieve goals without a plan, but the problem with plans is they never seem to work out the way we first envisage. This is because a plan is a series of assumptions about future events and anticipated activities – and none of us can see the future clearly. In fact, as soon as we decide on a goal, a quiet little inner voice is likely to point out a hundred obstacles to achieving it.

Unfortunately, conventional wisdom and what will work are often two different things. Some of the client case studies in this book are remarkable simply because of the way these individuals challenged conventional wisdom and changed it. The attitudes and beliefs of the individuals concerned allowed them to ask questions and take steps to organise their own rehabilitation. They didn't accept that things could not be better, instead setting out to make 'better' their reality; but not everyone is going to adjust to life after a spinal cord injury like Christopher Reeve, Mark Pollock or Claire Lomas. Some will need a little help in the personal attitude and belief department.

There is a martial arts principle of blending with the forces of life. If we use it, we can save ourselves a great deal of pain. There are four ways to approach the forces of life:

1. Surrender to them fatalistically but accept the consequences.

2. Ignore them, but the consequence is still to struggle against the natural currents of life.

3. Resist them and create turmoil, wasting energy and fighting ourselves.

4. Use them and blend with nature – the principle of non-resistance. Like birds that ride the wind,

people too can make use of the natural forces of life.

Notice how you can make a choice. Once upon a time, it was fashionable to say that all you had to do was believe in yourself and anything would be possible. Sorry – this is not true. What is true is that you can strive to make improvements.

The placebo effect

Let's look at the strange benefits that flow from something called the placebo effect. A placebo is a substance or treatment that is designed to have no therapeutic value. Even back in 1931, researchers recognised that the placebo effect was a useful model to better understand the safety and efficacy of medicines in development (Walach, 2011). In other words, some patients would say that they felt better after the suggestion that they were being given a remedy.

Researchers in 1931 were interested in measuring the effects of a drug called sanocrysin on patients with tuberculosis and wanted to discount this observable placebo effect (Walach, 2011). Their idea was to give some patients a glass of distilled water while telling them they were really receiving sanocrysin.

It's reasonable to think that a placebo only works because the person receiving it doesn't know it's a placebo. Actually, it works because of belief. In his book *Time for a Change*, Richard Bandler (1993) describes (tongue in cheek) how he and a graduate student planned to market placebo pills to the public. A person would look up 'Headaches', for example, in the index they provided and find that placebos worked five times out of six when tested against other drugs.

The USA's drug regulatory body, the FDA, complained that the effects would wear off and the placebo would lose its efficacy. Bandler knew that this could happen because some people would not have strong enough beliefs first time around, so revealed his back-up plan: 'Placebo Plus, twice as powerful as before'.

If the basis of placebo is belief, we must have learned or adopted that belief in some way. If all beliefs are learned, we can also change or 'unlearn' them. Essentially, beliefs are nothing to do with facts; they are a mental construct of an individual or a group of individuals. We can distinguish between placebo and the placebo effect. Basically, any sort of treatment can act as a placebo, but what determines the placebo effect is the actual response of the patient to the intervention.

One of the most enduring questions about the placebo effect is whether this is an effect of human physiology or psychology: is it of the mind or the body? Research is now demonstrating that it is both. As we have already seen, modern thinking recognises that mind and body are not separate entities and what happens with one always affects the other (Pert, 1997).

Research at the Harvard Medical School (Kaptchuk and Miller, 2015) is showing that a change in the mindset or attitude of a patient alters their neurochemistry. Patients affected by pain and debility look to doctors and allied health professionals for the words, gestures and deeds that reinforce their belief in medicine's power and their expectation that they will benefit from an intervention. The neurochemical changes they experience from a change of mindset have a catalytic effect on many of their body systems.

Belief, attitude and expectation – we could label these as contributors to hope – can be embedded and shaped by the encounter between patient and medical expert. This hope produces an effect that can block pain by releasing endorphins and enkephalins, which in turn influence fundamental processes such as respiration, circulation, elimination and motor function. Hope is the leverage that can start a cascade of physical effects, making improvement much more likely.

Doing as you are told

Sometimes, it is useful to sort out how we as people are motivated. Fundamentally, we all tend to be motivated by moving towards pleasure or away from pain, but there are many more moving away from pain people than those actively moving towards pleasure. In other words, there are more people running away from a threat than approaching a future aim.

Let's have a look at Mrs Smith. She is a moving away from pain patient. When you want to attract her with positive benefits such as better mobility or improved core strength, it simply won't work. For her, new treatment would only seem like gold if she knew it would help her avoid some dire consequence – and remember that what would be a dire outcome for Mrs Smith may not be so for you. It's the individual's perception that matters.

Mrs Jones, by contrast, is a moving towards pleasure patient. She would not be motivated by the same things as Mrs Smith; she would be much more interested in the fact that a new treatment may mean she can go to her daughter's wedding or stay independent into old age.

If you know how someone is motivated, you avoid having to struggle against their will when they simply do not see the world the way you do. This works with doctors, therapists, assistants – everyone, even your children.

How do you find out if someone is an away from pain or towards pleasure person? I suggest you don't interrogate them, but instead get to know them by asking about certain situations and seeing how they respond. By looking to compare or contrast their responses with how you would react, you can easily see what will work for them.

Why not start with yourself? Go back to a time in your life when you were strongly motivated to do something and took action. Remember what it felt like. What did you see, hear, feel? For contrast, think of a situation where you knew that you needed to do something, but you procrastinated. You waited and waited until the pain of further delay overcame your resistance to act. Note again what you saw, heard and felt.

All I can tell you is that getting someone to act (including you yourself) is much easier if you are working with representations that motivate them rather than ones that lead to procrastination. Take opportunities to adapt these representations so that you get the responses you want in yourself and other people.

KEY POINT

What's the lesson here? My one-time mentor Michael Breen pointed out that if you are going to have beliefs, make sure they are useful ones. This is relevant to your rehabilitation journey when the words and actions of those around you can lift you up and give you a base to move forward, or extinguish your hope.

Summary

A spinal cord injury doesn't just affect our body – it undermines a belief structure founded on an illusion that we will have control of our path through life. This kind of catastrophic injury sooner or later reminds us of two uncomfortable things:

ASSORTED MIND GAMES

- At some point, we will be alone or abandoned.
- We must inevitably lose control of reality.

Clients have often said to me that their doctor killed hope by encouraging them to be realistic about their goals and plans. The truth is we all like and need hope, but we should not allow others to be its source. We have to make hope our choice because choice is the only thing we truly have control over. Like it or not, we are all playing mind games and at stake is our quality of life.

Athletes and high performers in life seem to choose at will to adopt a mindset that leads to success, but the difference between success and failure is often as thin as a razor's edge. These high performers are not so different from you or me. We can all learn this skill.

One of the simplest ways to a more resourceful state is to influence the way we breathe. The breath has a powerful effect on our heart and our ANS. When we power our breath with feelings, we send a signal to our brain that leads to clarity of thought. This gets us out of helplessness.

Learning to adopt a resourceful mindset is vital to your quality of life because it determines the behaviours that will be possible for you. These in turn produce your results. Choose your weapons wisely.

Claire Lomas's story

Claire's passion was horse riding and eventing. A talented and high-level rider, she had a bad fall at Osberton Horse Trials in May 2007 and experienced a T4 spinal cord injury. She received initial treatment at Queen's Medical Centre in Nottingham where doctors told her that it was highly unlikely she would walk again. She describes her early days in intensive care in detail in her first book, *Finding My Feet* (Lomas, 2014): 'Two-thirds of me was dead. My breathing was getting worse, and I was put on a ventilator.'

Thanks to pneumonia, her early days in hospital were a blur, but she described her time in intensive care as 'something special'. Then came the upheaval of transfer to the Sheffield Spinal Injury Unit where rehabilitation could begin.

Claire wrote:

> 'There were two ways of looking at things: I was having the worst time I could ever imagine, or I was extremely lucky. It was also a journey that made me a better person, but of course I didn't know that at the time.'

Unfortunately, the physiotherapy she was getting was not what she expected. Sessions were limited to three per week for forty-five minutes and gave her no inspiration to improve. It seemed to Claire that everything was targeted towards her accepting her level of disability. Any talk of recovering movement or sensation was treated as her being in denial or having false hope. In fact, Claire knew the severity of her injury, but saw real value in having hope and positive expectation.

I met Claire at her home after discharge. She had a treadmill, hoist and harness set up in the garage, and I introduced her to FES cycling which she now uses frequently as part of her exercise regime. At that first visit, I had no idea about what her future exploits would be. I remember her as a lovely and enthusiastic person, typical of the sportspeople I have met, in her willingness to seek to challenge herself.

Claire chose to do the London Marathon in an exoskeleton in 2012 as a vehicle to raise funds for spinal cord injury research. Completing the distance of the London Marathon took her seventeen days to achieve. Little did we know that this wasn't to be the last of her adventures; to date, she has raised over £825,000 for charity and has been awarded an MBE.

She particularly impressed me by seeking and obtaining a motorcycle race licence, despite her paralysis. Her original idea of doing a parade lap at the Isle of Man TT has not been allowed by the organisers to date – I doubt she has given up on that one – but obtaining her pilot's licence might be some consolation. Many companies have chosen to listen to Claire's story at corporate events – she's a truly inspirational lady.

In Claire's second book, *The Bigger Picture*, she describes much more of her personal attitudes to life, and I recommend it to you. Many statements in this book jump out, but one I particularly like is this: 'We can begin something without knowing where exactly we are going. Just make sure you do start though' (Lomas, 2022).

You can learn more about Claire's story at www.claireschallenge.co.uk

FOUR
The Rehabilitation Journey

So far in Part One, we've looked at what happens immediately after a catastrophic injury and the weeks or months that follow while the injured person is still hospitalised or in a specialist unit, but there comes a time when that person will have to regain their independence. In this chapter, we will look at how to prepare for the return home.

No one chooses to have their life turned upside down, but there are practical considerations that anyone with a spinal cord injury will have to consider as they think towards venturing back out into the world. Not least among those is how they're going to survive financially.

Injury and negligence

If you have suffered injury or illness because of someone else's negligence, you may be able to claim compensation and get practical help with rehabilitation to aid your recovery. If this is the case, it is advisable to get early advice from a specialist personal injury lawyer. In the UK, the Association of Personal Injury Lawyers (APIL) publishes a directory of providers and its 'Best Practice Guide on Rehabilitation', which are both good sources of information. The latter is aimed at professionals but can be generally useful.

It's important to get advice early as starting rehabilitation as soon as possible often leads to the best outcomes. The aim of rehabilitation is to restore the injured person to as productive and independent a lifestyle as possible, but this is often no simple task. Legal precedent in the UK has been in place since 1880 and has established that the purpose of damages is to restore the injured party to the position he or she would have been in if not for the negligence of the defendant.

In catastrophic-injury cases, a medical expert report will likely be commissioned to cover all aspects of care such as the need for therapy, housing, psychology, employment, specialist equipment and more. A case manager, who tends to have a background as a nurse, therapist or other clinical specialist, acts on behalf of the injured person to coordinate and establish the person's needs in a broad sense. A good case manager will have a range of relevant connections and knowledge to help coordinate the rehabilitation process, so they are a great resource, but may have several clients to look after. It's important to like and trust the one you work with as you may not always have their undivided attention.

In my experience, people who have suffered a spinal cord injury due to someone else's negligence really benefit from the skills personal injury lawyers can bring. Experience counts in this domain, so seek one with specialist knowledge of working with your particular injury. This may be new territory for you, but your legal team will then be able to draw on a wealth of practical experience. While monetary compensation would be a real help, the guidance and sense of normality that a good legal team can bring is of equal value.

KEY POINT

It is important to act quickly and identify a credible personal injury law firm. Seeking compensation for something that was not your fault is not an easy or quick path to take, so expert guidance is essential.

The home environment

One of the common reasons for delayed discharge from hospital is that the home environment is not suitable for the injured person to return to. Just recently, I visited a client and discovered I had to carry equipment from the street up nineteen steps to get to the front door. I was relieved to hear that they were moving to a new home; it's simply impossible for a disabled person to access that house as it is and there's no easy way of modifying the means of access.

In the same week, I had a call from someone wanting a product demonstration for his father. Unfortunately, the father was unable to come downstairs (the family was waiting – and waiting – for the installation of a lift) and I was unable to carry a 120 kg product up the stairs for the demonstration.

Such barriers are obvious, but the majority are more subtle. They're influenced by the nature of the person's injury and whether carers and specialist equipment are required. The best advice is to obtain an environmental assessment by a knowledgeable healthcare professional. Here are some of the issues that they will need to explore.

It is fundamental to check the access in and out of your house. Is there a need for a ramp? Is it level access into your house or do you need to cross a raised threshold, double-glazing door base or other potential barrier? Is there carpet or laminate flooring in your house? Is there a garden and can it be accessed?

Inside the house, there may be issues with the layout of rooms and their accessibility. I have visited clients who can no longer access the upstairs bedroom and are now faced with sleeping in a downstairs room; I have even seen beds in the kitchen. In general, there

THE REHABILITATION JOURNEY

are always going to be access issues and sometimes these can be dealt with by redesign.

Most kitchens are not designed for those in a wheelchair. I have had several clients choose to use a Tek RMD standing mobility device (see the 'Standing for health' section of Chapter Five) as it lets them access a standard kitchen as an alternative to redesigning the room.

It's not just a case of accessibility; it is important to understand what tasks you will need to carry out in the various rooms and which equipment will support you in these tasks. You may, for example, be able to self-transfer from wheelchair to bed, or you may need to be hoisted. Hoists can be portable or ceiling/wall mounted, which allows use in areas without much floor space. There are many hoist and sling types, so it is important to get the most suitable for your needs.

Using hoists is a topic that needs particular attention with a manual-handling risk assessment. This considers what type of tasks an individual will carry out, who is doing the hoisting (a family member or a care team) and the environment in which the hoisting takes place. Manual-handling professionals will refer to the acronym TILE – which stands for tasks, individuals, load (weight of the user) and environment – when considering these requirements.

Beds can be height adjustable and profiling, both of which can greatly ease transfers. Some people will need the bed to be accessible on both sides or may benefit from a bed with pressure management features.

What about the bathroom? It may be that you can have an adapted wet floor/shower area with toilet. On a similar subject, when you're out and about, check the national network of Changing Places (www.changing-places.org) for accessible toilets in public buildings.

> **KEY POINT**
>
> Many private therapy firms specialising in catastrophic injuries will have occupational therapists who can advise on adapting your home environment and making sure that essential equipment is in place.

The charity sector

Although I cannot describe all relevant charities nor do them justice in terms of the work they do, it is important to recognise the value they provide to people at this most difficult time in life. Charities have a variety of objectives, including generating political influence, offering a trusted community, providing counselling and advice, funding research, introducing people to sport, assisting with rehabilitation and simply inspiring others. You are likely to find it beneficial to reach out and connect with this network of support.

The charity that every spinal cord injured person is most likely to get to know is the Spinal Injury Association (SIA). Not every person who has a spinal

THE REHABILITATION JOURNEY

cord injury will be treated in a specialist centre and this will tend to delay or compromise their recovery. Organisations such as the SIA provide access to people and resources that can be vital.

The SIA's stated aim is to be the go-to place for everyone affected by spinal cord injury, so that they can quickly connect to the charity's vast network of people, organisations and services. This is a worthy but demanding remit. Find out more at www.spinal.co.uk.

One of my business's favourite charities is the Rooprai Spinal Trust (known as RST or RS Trust), which was established in 2005, inspired by Marrianne Rooprai who was paralysed from the shoulders down in the summer of 2004. Today, RST is a multi-award-winning charity that has an ever-expanding group of supporters from around the world. With no staffing costs or office rentals, it prides itself on being a modern, forward-thinking, streamlined organisation.

One of RST's innovative activities is to fund physiotherapy scholarships. The supporters of the charity are massive believers in the power of exercise following a spinal cord injury and have established a programme to guide people to tap into this power, learn how to set goals and keep complications at bay. Marrianne features in many of the exercise videos and is incredibly inspiring. She has a high-level cervical injury, but constantly challenges expectations with her physical achievements.

Find out more at www.rstrust.com.

The Matt Hampson Foundation was created to support young people seriously injured through sport. Matt Hampson OBE was a top-level rugby player, but his life changed dramatically in 2005 when a scrum collapsed causing a high-level spinal cord injury. From being an independent England and Leicester Tigers prospect, he ended up needing round-the-clock care.

The Foundation's aim is to provide advice, support, relief and treatment for anyone suffering serious injury or disability that has primarily arisen from participation in or training for any sport or sporting activity. It recently opened the Get Busy Living Centre, which serves as both a social space and gym equipped and staffed to suit this clientele. Situated in a beautiful spot near Melton Mowbray, Leicestershire, this facility is impressive.

Find out more about the Matt Hampson Foundation at www.matthampsonfoundation.org.

KEY POINT

When something as life changing as a catastrophic injury happens to you, it can be easy to end up feeling isolated. The charities I have mentioned here are among many that will help you to find a network of support invaluable to your sense of wellbeing and purpose.

The purpose of rehabilitation

The purpose of rehabilitation is to restore an injured person to as productive and independent a lifestyle as possible using appropriately timed medical, functional and vocational interventions. It sounds easy, but in fact can be immensely complex.

A spinal cord injury can disrupt many of the physical functions we take for granted and the individual nature of the injury to the spine will strongly influence what parts of the body are affected. This typically shapes the form of the treatment offered both early on and in subsequent rehabilitation.

There are always beliefs and expectations for recovery, some of which may be based on clinical anecdotes or evidence. Here are a few of the prevailing ones:

- People with a complete injury often can regain control of one or two levels of muscle movement.

- People with an incomplete injury are more likely to regain control of muscle movement than people with a complete injury.

- If you are seeing some improvement, like regaining muscle movement, it raises your chances for more improvement.

- The longer you go without seeing improvement, the lower your chances for improvement.

We must not make the mistake of assuming that these beliefs or paradigms for treatment are correct in some absolute sense. If that were the case, we would have to conclude that we can't expect any future improvements beyond these guidelines.

A rehabilitation approach that makes sense in theory (when resources are not constrained) is intensive exercise-based therapy to recover as much bodily function as possible (restitution), and then compensate with assistive devices and approaches for the functions that you cannot recover. The challenge is knowing where the boundary is between the imperatives of restitution and compensation. Once a patient is medically stable and the focus shifts to rehabilitation, the role of the therapist and other members of the clinic team is ideally to be like physical training instructors.

Claire Lomas described her experience of hospital rehabilitation to me as a less than uplifting experience at times. She could see all the equipment available for rehabilitation but was advised that there was little point in her using it unless her legs showed signs of recovery. The physiotherapy she received focused on the parts of her body that did work and neglected the paralysed parts. This might seem pragmatic in our world of scarce resources, but pragmatism can sometimes kill hope.

It is imperative to pursue restitution vigorously in the early weeks and months following injury because of the natural property of our body to seek stability of its processes. This is termed homeostasis, which is a fancy way of saying that the body always operates on the basis of 'use it or lose it' and will tend to adapt or compensate for functions that are lost. Although some potential for functional improvement will remain for years, delays to restitution tend to make recovery more complex and expensive to achieve. Bodily compensations for the primary injury can greatly complicate attempts to recover function. In fact, they can make it difficult to identify the core problem.

In the UK, we are very lucky to have the NHS that promises to provide care for free at the point of delivery. Many of us grew up believing that the NHS would always be there for us if we ever needed it, but now our population is ageing. Although people are living longer than those of old, they are not necessarily healthier.

In all the so-called developed economies, we are seeing many people succumb to chronic conditions that damage their quality of life and place significant and unsustainable economic pressure on society. Many individuals survive a health crisis, such as a spinal cord injury, but then need support and care for the rest of their lives. The resources available to support the NHS and the related social services are never going to be sufficient to meet all expectations for rehabilitation and we are not likely to see this change for the better.

You can see the problem, I'm sure. There is only so much resource to go around and spinal cord injury rehabilitation in general will have to compete with other deserving cases for a share of the public purse. What most of us don't realise until it directly affects us or a family member, is that conditions such as spinal cord injury, which are catastrophic, inevitably challenge everything that we treasure about life.

The NHS is fantastic at acute care with processes and methods that are very effective, but it's less able to support us on our personal lifelong rehabilitation journey. In fact, the attention we get in hospital towards rehabilitation will be influenced by the medical profession's determination of what our potential for recovery might be. When resources are scarce, this makes rational sense, but there are times when we should challenge these judgements.

In recent years, people have frequently been discharged from hospital and described as having no potential for improvement. The reality is that there is almost always potential for improvement, but unfortunately the state cannot provide the resources to pursue this any longer.

KEY POINT

If you are discharged from hospital with no further potential for improvement, it may be that lack of resources is the driver behind this assessment. As long as you don't compromise your safety, it may be worthwhile challenging this assessment, even when it comes from the medical profession. This is another area where the charities I mentioned earlier can help.

Neuroplasticity

Neuroplasticity is a term that is often used (and sometimes misused) today. It points to the fact that neurological body systems can be provoked to adapt, recover and learn new functions even many years after an injury.

While spinal cord injuries can result in a vast array of functional deficits, many of which are life threatening, most of these injuries are anatomically incomplete as we learned in Chapter One. This fact and the recognition of neuroplasticity have given rise to much optimism about the prospects for functional gains in rehabilitation, far beyond what we previously might have expected.

Neuroplasticity is defined as the potential for functional and anatomical changes of the nervous system in response to stimuli during learning or in response to injury (Kandel et al, 2013). In other words, it's about the central nervous system's apparent ability to rewire its neural circuitry to make adaptive changes. It might in some circumstances allow for functions affected by spinal cord injury to be relearned and recovered. In popular literature, neuroplasticity is generally looked upon as a positive thing, but we will see why this is not always the case.

When we walk, two sources of information are processed by the spinal cord. One comes from above: instructions from the brain about where we want to go based on what we see. The other comes from below: sensory information from the muscles, tendons and skin. After a spinal cord injury, the communication lines between the brain and body are cut or dramatically diminished, depending on the severity of the event.

Doctors and researchers once thought it impossible for us to regain any type of control over the limbs without instructions from the brain, but unlike fixed mechanical circuits, the brain and spinal cord, as it turns out, are malleable. Connections between neurons grow or atrophy based on activity.

The Dalai Lama watched a brain operation during a visit to an American medical school in the early 1990s. Since the 1980s, neuroscientists had understood that mental experiences reflect both chemical and electrical changes in the brain – when electrical impulses pass through our visual cortex, for instance, we see; when neurochemicals course through the limbic system, we feel.

The Dalai Lama knew this explanation, but something had always bothered him about it, so he asked if it could work the other way around. As well as the brain giving rise to thoughts and hopes and beliefs and emotions that add up to the thing we call the mind, maybe the mind could act back on the brain and body to cause physical changes in the very matter that created it. If so, then pure thought would change the brain's activity, its circuits or even its structure.

At the time, one brain surgeon confidently asserted that physical states give rise to mental states, but 'downward' causation – from the mental to the physical – was not possible. Despite this slap down, though, the Dalai Lama had put his finger on an emerging revolution in brain research. Neuroscientists have since overthrown the age-old dogma that the adult brain can't change.

The relatively recent exciting discovery that the nervous system is plastic and adaptable even in adulthood is a source of great hope to people with spinal cord injury and other disorders of the central nervous system such as stroke. We now call this ability neuroplasticity. Its discovery has led to promising new treatments for a range of conditions and as we learn more, neuroplasticity should continue to lead to progress in rehabilitation.

The basic idea is that if we can practise a movement in a particular way, we might recover lost function at least in part. For example, a person whose arm movement is affected by stroke might be able to recover useful function providing they can practise the required movement often enough. The flip side of this is we must 'use it or lose it'.

Currently, repeated practice and specific training provide the best opportunities to reverse the maladaptive plasticity associated with neuropathology and promote instead the adaptive plasticity supportive of function. We can become a victim of the nervous system's plasticity if we don't act to take advantage of it, but much is still unknown about how to optimise this.

We could think of neuroplasticity as learning dependent – a process of applying a stimulus and getting a beneficial outcome as a result. Evidence suggests that several non-invasive clinically accessible forms of energy can be a source of useful stimulus (Robertson et al, 2006). Electrical, magnetic and vibration stimuli may be used to augment the effects of training.

In essence, stimulation activates the same neural circuits that are activated by training, and when used in combination with training, stimulation has the potential to promote neuroplasticity beyond that achieved by practice or training alone. Studies involving neurologically healthy individuals have shown these approaches to enhance neural excitability and motor performance. Non-invasive clinically available forms of stimulation may be used to modulate neural excitability as an adjuvant to programmes designed to improve hand/arm or walking function in people with neurological disorders. I will describe examples of this in Chapter Six.

There are several factors commonly involved in motor learning and hence neuroplasticity. To some extent, they overlap:

- Carrying out a skill practice that is challenging, but not too difficult.
- Practice should be specific.
- Skill practice must be intense.
- Practice should be progressive.
- Timing matters.
- Engage motivation to enhance the learning.

Let's describe each of these in more detail.

Research evidence shows that the difficulty of the task matters to the process of learning (Magness, 2022). The challenge is how to create a situation where practice is difficult and cognitively engaging, but not impossible.

Specificity effects have been recognised in learning research for more than 100 years, the general finding being that transfer of skills from practice to real-world application will be small unless the skills required are nearly identical. What this means is that general exercise and activities like strength training are most effective when combined with task-specific training programmes. Research is now looking at how practice in one task can transfer to another task in a meaningful way.

What do we mean by 'intense'? Intensity implies that some combination of the dose, frequency and duration of training practice is important to getting results. Although this suggestion is supported by research results, there is a lack of detail when we try to pin down what exactly is a necessary and sufficient level of intensity for an individual case.

Some researchers point out that being able to tap into someone's motivation to practise may be more effective than simply cranking up the intensity of the practice. The idea here is that focusing on practice simply to reduce impairment is less motivating than looking at seeking benefits that directly impact on the person's quality of life.

There is no doubt that repeated attempts to solve a motor-control task benefit neuroplasticity and motor learning, but tasks must not be too simple or repetitive. Simple tasks well within the capability of the performer will not induce neural plasticity. What's needed could be described as 'repetition without repetition'.

Imagine learning a golf swing that involves lots of repetition. Let's say you have been taught well and don't see learning the golf swing as just rapidly hitting 1,000 golf balls down the driving range. For each stroke, you learn to follow the same thoughtful process with careful setup and attention to detail. However carefully you try to replicate each golf swing, there are going to be lots of small deviations in muscle and limb joint activity, and so on. What seems like exact repetition is not exactly so, but over time, you may consciously learn from your results and refine your swing.

When it comes to robotic systems that allow repetitive practice, perhaps the same observations hold. For example, the Icone robot for upper-limb rehabilitation allows the user to practise arm movement guided within an adjustable 'haptic tunnel'. This allows the task to take place repetitively without constraining the movement to be the same with each repetition. Over time, the haptic tunnel's size can be adjusted as the user's performance improves.

Different forms of plasticity occur at different times during training. This implies that the timing of an intense therapy programme is important. Some researchers are advocating early interventions, for example in the first month after a stroke. This seems to make sense, but a lot of stroke research has only been carried out in the chronic phase of recovery. Many therapeutic interventions rely on extrinsic motivation to be effective. It seems to me that the best results come when motivation is intrinsic and the person's mindset is adjusted to provide a consistent drive to work at improvement. In Chapter Five, we will look at neuroplasticity in the context of training and exercise to tap into this phenomenon.

KEY POINT

Neuroplasticity is a natural process that we can take advantage of or suffer the consequences. It can be the source of potential improvement in function, but if we do nothing, we will see the body's 'use it or lose it' process at work.

Goal setting in rehabilitation

Setting and achieving goals in any area of life can be a challenge. You have probably heard of the SMART acronym for rational goal setting, which stands for specific, measurable, achievable, realistic and time bound. While this is good general guidance for many business situations, there are often practical issues with parts of this recipe in rehabilitation after a spinal cord injury.

Whenever the stakes are high, it can be difficult to weigh up exactly what is achievable and realistic. Some people are more comfortable with audacious goals than others. When outcomes depend on certain things outside of our control, this obviously compromises what we can achieve, but this book is about maximising potential.

Goal setting between clinicians and their clients is a complex and emotional, but fundamental part of rehabilitation. The good news is that neuroplasticity is real and suggests that the potential for motor learning and some physical recovery may not have been totally extinguished by a catastrophic injury. The bad news is that we do not necessarily know the most effective ways of activating neuroplasticity and adapting it to the needs of everyone.

Goal setting directs rehabilitation interventions towards a specific outcome or outcomes that result in improved recovery – if it's managed skilfully. Shared goal setting can also help to coordinate members of a multidisciplinary team and ensure they are working together towards a common goal and don't miss anything. Thirdly, goals can be used to evaluate the success of rehabilitation interventions.

Professor in neurological rehabilitation at Oxford University, Derick Wade, has provided an evidence-based description of effective rehabilitation. His paper (Wade, 2020) suggests that rehabilitation may benefit anyone with a long-term disability, however that disability has come about, at any stage and any age, in any setting. To be effective, rehabilitation depends on a multidisciplinary team of experts working towards shared goals.

We would all, I'm sure, like to think that clinicians will always know exactly what rehabilitation their patients can achieve and how to communicate this clearly to their patients, who could then see this as a meaningful goal they can commit to. Unfortunately, this is never going to be the case. Clinicians often cannot know exactly what the injured person can achieve. Wade goes on to say a huge range of other interventions may be needed in rehabilitation, making it an extremely complex process. Specific actions must be tailored to the needs, goals and wishes of the individual patient, but the consequences remain unpredictable.

KEY POINT

Goals always need to be meaningful to the injured person, as those who are driven to succeed will make greater progress than those who are not.

Summary

Rehabilitation after a spinal cord injury is a journey that takes careful planning and commitment. Some people may have the help and guidance of a case manager and specialist legal team; if this applies to you, remember that they are *your* advisors and you need to be at the centre of everything that happens.

Rehabilitation is about restoring the injured person to as productive and independent a lifestyle as possible. The goals that the injured person sets with their rehabilitation team are individual to the patient, but likely to be shaped by everybody's beliefs about what is possible based on the nature of the injury and the resources available. There has never been a time in history to be more optimistic about the potential to maximise recovery thanks to our growing knowledge of neuroplasticity, technology and intensive rehabilitation.

When the time comes for the injured person to leave hospital or a specialist unit, the home environment and its suitability need careful professional attention. If it's unsuitable, your home environment will delay your discharge from hospital, so this is something to consider carefully as early as possible.

Dan Eley's story

Dan Eley worked as a teacher in Surrey and an outreach worker in Colombia before suffering a spinal cord injury in a diving accident while on holiday with friends in the Amazon in 2010. His injuries were life changing, leaving him paralysed from the shoulders downwards.

As I'm sure you can imagine, the Amazon is not ambulance friendly, so Dan's evacuation was not easy. Prolonged contact with a stretcher led to severe pressure ulcers and a risk to his life. Dan spent one year in hospital, initially fighting for his life, and then facing up to the enormous physical and emotional challenges of being so severely paralysed.

After leaving hospital, Dan was looking for a new purpose to rebuild his life. Drawing on his experience as a teacher and outreach worker, he decided to start a charity to help enable disadvantaged young people to access vocational training and be supported to find employment.

The Dan Eley Foundation (DEF) runs a project with a grassroots partner charity in Colombia called Fundación Educación para Todos (FEDUT). DEF and FEDUT run technical training courses for young people from marginalised urban areas in the city of Cali, and also operate as a recruitment agency, helping to match graduates to employment vacancies in local companies.

Since the start of its alliance with FEDUT in 2012, DEF has trained over 700 students as accountancy and marketing apprentices. Many of the course graduates are now working in gainful employment, providing more economic security for them and their families. Since 2016, the charity has been concentrating on disadvantaged young people locally in Surrey, the focus being on sponsoring specific individuals to undertake extracurricular activities, excursions, activities and/or training opportunities that facilitate personal development. DEF has supported approximately 400 young people through such interventions to date. During the Covid-19 pandemic, DEF provided financial assistance to four schools in Surrey, including donating laptops and funding interactive whiteboards for classrooms, to help individual students obtain and access vital educational materials and services.

Dan has also been able to draw on his experience of overcoming adversity to deliver motivational speeches as a keynote speaker. In 2012, Dan was chosen as a torchbearer for the London Olympics and had the privilege of carrying the torch on the high street of his hometown, Godalming.

Dan hopes his life experience will inspire youngsters to believe in themselves and that they can make a success of their lives, despite personal obstacles. You can read more about Dan's work at http://daneleyfoundation.org.

PART TWO
LONG-TERM HEALTH

In this part, we are going to look at approaches to building resilience and avoiding complications. In Chapter Two, we saw that the average life-span expectation for people after a spinal cord injury is pretty much the same as for the general population, but are you content to be average? You can choose instead to strive for improved quality of life and long-term fitness.

How do you achieve this? In this part, we will examine some of the approaches and technologies that are being used to promote long-term health and functional recovery for people with a spinal cord injury. Perhaps the oldest and most practical technology for health is exercise in its various forms – and this is something that everyone needs. Whatever the level of injury, exercise is medicine, so in this part we look at how best to get it. Perhaps surprising to some people is the fact that one of the simplest exercises we can do is to stand.

FES cycling and exoskeletons feature in this part, along with a look at orthotic bracing and other more common therapy and assistive technology. We will also look at nutrition which, alongside exercise, is vital for health. Finally, we'll consider emerging research which shows promise in pushing back the frontiers of knowledge about spinal cord injury.

FIVE
Fit For Life

The three major factors that influence our health and longevity are genetics, the environment (including nutrition) and our behaviour (Sallis, 2009). Because we have little control over genetic factors, it is critical that we focus on the environmental and behavioural factors we can control to improve health. In any event, research is now showing that our inherited genetics have less to do with our expectations for health than we once thought (Hofmekler, 2017).

Physical inactivity in the general population has become perhaps the greatest public health problem of our time, so finding a way to get everyone more active is critical to improving health and longevity in the twenty-first century. The beneficial relationship between exercise and health has been well known since the fifth century BCE, when Hippocrates said,

'Eating alone will not keep a man well; he must also take exercise. For food and exercise ... work together to produce health', and years of scientific research show a clear correlation between physical activity and health status. Unfortunately, this knowledge hasn't yet resulted in the healthcare system fully embracing exercise as a key prevention of illness.

Exercise is medicine

In general terms, it is tragic that so little has been done to address the one major factor affecting our health and longevity that is almost entirely under our control. My friend and associate Andrew Galbraith put it well when he said, 'Take time for exercise or make time for sickness.' There is no doubt that exercise is medicine for everyone, but it has particular importance for people with a spinal cord injury that will limit the ease with which they can carry it out.

For any human being, sitting at a desk or in front of the television for protracted periods is associated with increased risk of disease and a shorter life span, even among people who also choose to exercise. Worldwide, physical inactivity is arguably on a par with smoking as a health risk, killing more than five million people annually. A research study of Scottish adults showed those watching more than two hours' worth of television a day had a 125% increase in cardiac events such as heart attack or stroke (Scientific American, 2018). A study of Australian adults reported that every hour

FIT FOR LIFE

accumulated watching television shortened life expectancy by twenty-two minutes (Scientific American, 2018).

Think about the influence of TV watching. I will save you the maths: bingeing *Game of Thrones* in its entirety – apparently more than sixty-three hours of content – will cost you one day on this planet. The key takeaway here is that none of us should think of exercise as optional – it is essential for our health. It's basically the way humans have evolved.

A classic way of designing an exercise plan is the frequency, intensity, time and type approach. This approach considers four basic elements of exercise – the frequency, intensity, time and type – as it is the combination and variation of these things that lead to greatest fitness.

Don't interpret this to mean that you have to take exercise to excess; as in most things in life, it's about finding the right balance. Millions of people around the world run long distances, whether in search of improved fitness or to burn calories and lose weight. You might think that they are always super fit, yet a recent review of competitive long-distance runners shows that they die at much the same rates as sedentary people (Thijs, 2016). Endurance athletes tend to produce a high level of stress in their bodies that can be damaging to health rather than restorative. Exercise is good, but this does not necessarily mean continually increasing your level of exercise.

Where paralysis affecting the limbs is complete, there are obvious limitations to how a person can exercise, and this is where technology can help. In the next chapter, we will look in detail at technology like FES cycling or even electrotherapy, which can sometimes allow active exercise of the muscles even when a person is paralysed and has no conscious ability to move the legs or arms for themselves. With incomplete injuries, there may be limited movement, but greater potential for exercise and technology to help restore function.

Your body adapts to what you get it to do on a regular basis. If you are inactive, muscle strength and condition will decline. Inactivity has metabolic consequences too and can lead to excess weight, diabetes and other undesirable effects. The right kind of activity restores strength and conditioning.

Neuroplasticity holds out hope that some recovery can be possible, even many years after a spinal cord injury. The 'recipe' for regaining functional movement is often described as carrying out exercise that is task specific, intensive and frequent. Unfortunately, this doesn't give us much to go on when it comes to devising a specific training programme for an individual with a spinal cord injury.

The body, when exposed to stimulus such as exercise, will adapt to that stimulus if it is presented often enough and with sufficient intensity. It is our whole nervous system that adapts, not just our muscles – it's our brain, nerves, bones, ligaments, muscles and so on. Exercise guidelines for adults with a spinal cord injury have been published by The University of British Columbia along with Loughborough

University (Ginnis et al, 2018). The aim of these guidelines is to suggest minimum thresholds for achieving improved cardiorespiratory fitness, muscle strength and cardio-metabolic health. For cardiorespiratory fitness and muscle strength benefits, adults with a spinal cord injury should engage in twenty minutes of moderate- to vigorous-intensity aerobic exercise twice per week, plus three sets of strength-training exercises for each major functioning muscle group at a moderate to vigorous intensity twice per week.

Shortly, we are going to draw on my knowledge of strength and conditioning training to suggest principles to consider. We will also look at a recent trend to set up intensive-therapy centres that place a heavy emphasis on technology. First, though, let's recognise a form of exercise that every person with a spinal cord injury is encouraged to do.

KEY POINT

We should not regard exercise as optional – it is essential for health in all of us.

Standing for health

You may not think of standing as a form of exercise, but it is both effective and practical for most people. Those who cannot walk or stand unaided due to a spinal cord injury must often sit for more than eight hours a day, and as a result are at risk of secondary complications including the development of pressure ulcers, limb contractures, weakened bones, compromised circulation and blood pressure, and aggravated bowel and bladder function.

While interventions such as physical therapy, specialist seating cushions, muscle stimulation etc can mitigate some of these complications, regular standing appears to be a practical preventative step that most people can take following a spinal cord injury. An improved sense of wellbeing and quality of life is associated with standing. Standing instead of sitting causes muscles to produce enzymes that help to clear fat from circulating blood.

For all of these reasons, clinicians encourage passive standing as soon as a spinal cord injured person's rehabilitation starts. This is aided by a product or structure that can typically stabilise at least the hips, knees and ankles. They vary with the level of injury, but these products tend to include so-called standing frames, standing wheelchairs and orthoses. A low-level incomplete spinal cord injury may make orthotic interventions, such as a knee-ankle-foot orthosis (KAFO), practical. Higher-level injuries, such as cervical or thoracic, will generally require support for the trunk as well as the legs when the injured person is standing.

Supported standing programmes have been integrated into clinical practice for over fifty years. All spinal cord injured people should be individually assessed for the potential benefits of standing, which are generally dependent on the injury presentation (level of injury to the spine), time since injury and patient preferences. Evidence-based guidelines define how long or how often adults with spinal cord injury need to stand (MASCIP, 2013). Paleg and Livingstone (2015) reviewed the literature and noted that stronger evidence underpins the impact of regular standing programmes on a range of motion and activity for both stroke and spinal cord injury populations with some mixed evidence supporting impact on bone-mineral density. Evidence for other outcomes is weak.

When health is our goal, resilience is a worthwhile outcome. To think of the qualities of resilience and the benefits of simply standing, we could do worse than imagine a tree. It stands rooted to the Earth yet is strong and flexible. It endures come what may, even though it doesn't move.

We all tend to think of strength in a way that is shaped by our culture, but it's interesting to look at other cultures to see how they cultivate health and strength by exercise. I have a long interest in the martial arts and discovered that in ancient times, anyone who wanted to learn combat martial arts in China had to learn something called Chi Kung first, which was about developing internal energy before building strong muscles. The technique, which was sometimes called 'standing like a tree', involves holding certain standing postures with knees flexed to some degree, arms raised and held out as if you're holding a large ball, and shoulders relaxed.

In most conventional exercise practised in the West, the emphasis is on intensity and getting your heart beating faster. Of course, this works; over time, you will get stronger and fitter, but you will find that before the body is tired, you are often limited by your heart rate and breathing. Many people find this hard and give up long before they can enjoy the benefits of exercise.

Chinese combat science commenced basic training with compulsory standing like a tree for a couple of years, because this exercises the muscular and vascular system while keeping the pulse rate within normal range and allowing comfortable breathing. It's easy to dismiss this as not demanding enough until you try it; from personal experience, I know it can be brutal. As a karate student, I was encouraged to hold a particular posture for up to twenty minutes, but when I was a beginner, I would not make it past two minutes.

The interested reader can find out more about this form of exercise by reading *The Way of Energy* (Lam, 1991) or *Empty Force* (Dong and Raffill, 1996).

Research for conventional standing suggests that a spinal cord injured person needs to use a standing device for thirty minutes, five times a week for positive impact on most outcomes such as self-care and standing balance, and joint ranges of motion, cardiorespiratory, strength, spasticity, pain, skin, and bladder and bowel function. Sixty minutes for four to six times a week may be required for positive impact on bone-mineral density and mental function (Paleg and Livingstone, 2015). While therapists can recommend with some confidence the use of a supported standing intervention to impact on preserving a joint range of motion and activity outcomes, the evidence is less certain for other outcomes. It makes sense, therefore, to measure outcomes for each spinal cord injured person to ensure effectiveness for individuals.

The most popular product in the UK is perhaps the standing frame, such as the wooden Oswestry or the more modern EasyStand designs. These achieve the basic objective of allowing a person with lower-limb paralysis to stand and may also allow other activities to take place at the same time. They need to be set up for the stature of the individual and made as easy and safe as possible for the spinal cord injured person to transfer on and off. The biggest issue I hear from clients is that they can take up too much space in modern houses and are a bit boring to use. 'Boring' is not exactly an incentive for regular use.

Standing wheelchairs have the advantage of allowing easy and frequent use as they combine two needs: the person can move around and stand when they want to with power assistance. There are even specialist powered chairs for activities such as golf. Being mobile is a big positive benefit, although standing wheelchairs do tend to have a large wheelbase and the standing posture will typically be inclined back to some extent to maintain stability. For this reason, they tend not to be the most useful products for prolonged standing.

People with an incomplete injury and some sufficiently preserved necessary muscle function may use KAFOs or other non-powered orthotic products. Modern materials such as carbon fibre have reduced the overall encumbrance of these products due to weight, but they involve a need for the injured person to use a rollator/walker or forearm crutches, which means that the hands and arms are not free to participate in other activities.

Orthoses should be custom made to a model of the person's limbs to avoid problems of pressure or rubs at the tissue interface. Conventional orthoses tend to be passive structures with joints, at least at the knee, which are locked during gait and unlocked when the user is seated. Some KAFOs can have knee joints that automatically lock and unlock via electromechanical means, but these are less frequently seen.

Exoskeletons and powered orthoses may extend their value to certain individuals, but their cost will put them out of reach for many. The repetitive impact loading generated by gait training in any orthosis or exoskeleton that puts the user directly in touch with the ground may lead to greater benefits in terms of bone-mineral density and bowel and bladder function when compared with other approaches to standing. We will cover orthotic products and exoskeletons in more detail in Chapter Six.

A less well-known technology-assisted method of standing is the Tek RMD from Matia Robotics. It is neither a standing wheelchair nor a passive standing device, but a unique product that allows users with a spinal cord or other neurological injury resulting in lower-limb paralysis or weakness to stand and move readily in an indoor or outdoor environment. The user of the Tek RMD largely has hands free to engage with their environment.

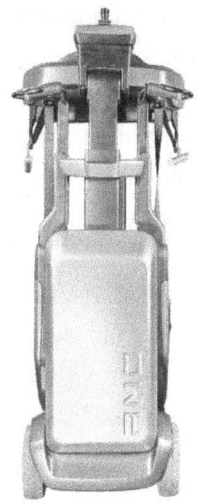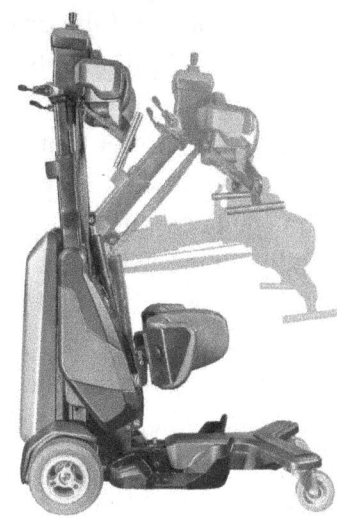

Tek RMD device
(illustration used with kind
permission of Matia Mobility)

Unlike the typical standing wheelchair, the Tek RMD does not tilt the user back when they're standing upright, so most users can achieve and hold a good therapeutic posture for long periods. Thick pads positioned just below the knee and at the chest and a seat cushion spanning the hip area enable the user to be held safely, whether they're fully upright, seated or at any point in between. This balanced posture allows them much easier interaction with the environment; many users find that they can at last use a standard kitchen layout and move at will from selecting something from a high shelf to accessing a low cupboard.

Each Tek RMD is set up to suit the stature of the individual user. Some people need more trunk support initially and the product can be reconfigured as the user's requirements change over time. What surprises many of my clients is that the product is both narrower and shorter than the typical wheelchair, so it is easy to manoeuvre. Using the control panel, the user may sit or stand and employ the joystick to steer around their environment.

The product is boarded from the back so users can transfer from a wheelchair, although this may depend upon the design of the chair and the person's transfer abilities. Others prefer to use a height-adjustable plinth or even a conventional chair for transfer. The manufacturer recently released a transfer seat which provides another alternative. It flips down for use and up for convenience when it's not needed.

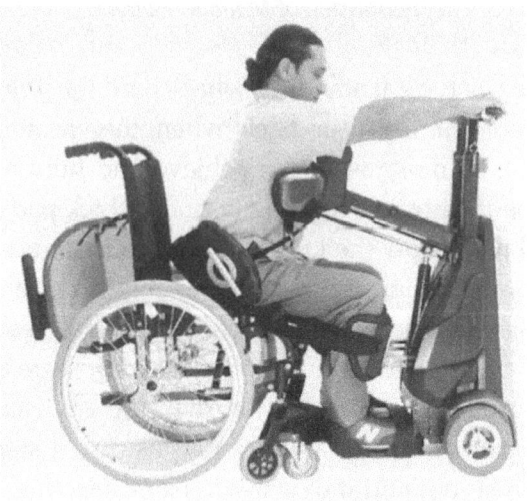

Tek RMD transfer
(illustration used with kind
permission of Matia Mobility)

FIT FOR LIFE

Once upright, the user can move around simply by using a joystick control. Initially envisaged as an indoor-use product, the Tek RMD now has outdoor wheels to make it suitable for grass and other surfaces. The kit allows users to change their product quickly and easily for indoor or outdoor use as the mood requires.

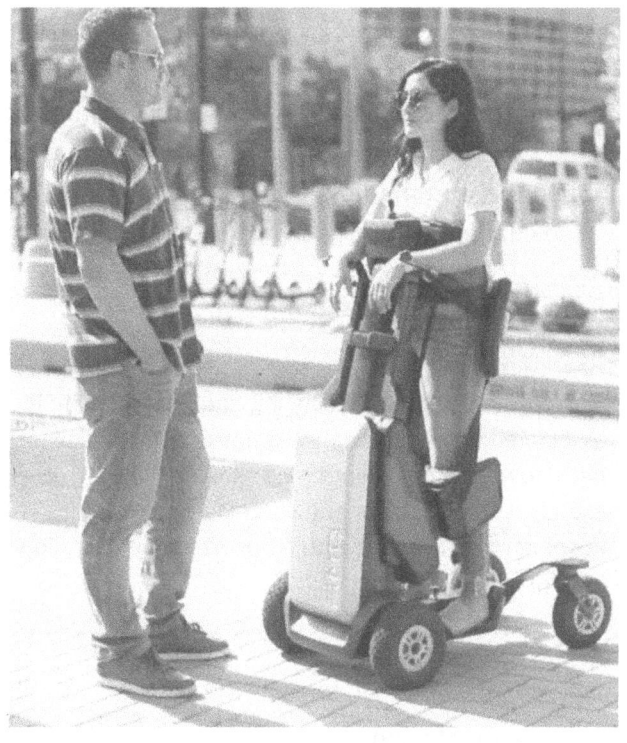

Out and about on a Tek RMD device
(illustration used with kind permission of Matia Mobility)

We can't ignore the cost of the technology with exoskeletons, standing wheelchairs and the Tek RMD being significantly more expensive than the purely standing options, but as the Tek RMD has allowed some users to return to work, they have been able to access some sources of public funding. Domestic users should find that they can achieve a good balance between social and therapeutic benefits.

It is always a good idea for people to understand that each product will have different strengths and weaknesses, and none can be perfect for everyone. As there are good clinical reasons to make standing part of life, I encourage you to weigh up the most suitable way of achieving this in your individual case. Establish the minimal level of support you need and strive to challenge your body.

KEY POINT

An improved sense of wellbeing and quality of life is associated with standing. As Chinese combat science has known since ancient times, standing like a tree exercises the muscular and vascular system while keeping the pulse rate within normal range and allowing comfortable breathing.

A low-cost alternative

Technology can provide a key to unlock progress in rehabilitation. There is no doubt about this, but sometimes people focus too much on looking for novel technology as the means and forget that it is getting results that counts. That shiny new piece of technology might be just what you need, but before you purchase it, reflect on exactly what it will contribute to your rehabilitation.

Most people who attend a gym are not competitive athletes and may have no definable objective other than losing a bit of weight and keeping fit. They are satisfied with simply exercising and the fitness industry is understandably attuned to this. Many modern health studios are typically laid out for exercising with half the floor space devoted to cardio equipment and the other half to machines designed primarily for the convenience of the users.

You can argue that machines make exercising safer, but they may not readily transfer into real-life utility. The places where real progress is made in strength and conditioning training have barbells, dumbbells and kettlebells. They have elastic cords and ropes with pulleys. In short, they have simple equipment that is unmatched to the floor space for building strength when exercise goals and progress matter. When I attended the Highland Games, where the focus is functional strength, the athletes worked with simple objects they could lift and throw. There was not an exercise machine in sight.

We should all be seeking out and making use of basic low-cost exercises for rehabilitation whenever we can. The standing like a tree process of ancient martial arts is an example: it's low-tech, simple and challenging, and it's free.

Your progress is not going to be eased by the amount you pay to exercise; we all have to do the best we can with the resources we have available. Technology might provide the means to exercise when this is impossible for you to do any other way, but make sure that you use the simple methods when you can. The most intensive exercise I have ever done is with a kettlebell, which is basically a heavy cannonball with a handle.

KEY POINT

You need to use some imagination to exercise when you have a spinal cord injury. Don't fall into the trap of thinking that expensive technology automatically means it'll be better than simple techniques humans have used for centuries to build strength.

Intensive rehabilitation centres

Around 2009, Peter Carr showed me what might have been the first UK facility dedicated to providing intensive rehabilitation for people following a spinal cord injury. The Standing Start organisation took root in Peter's back garden in Cambridgeshire in the form of a rather large shed stocked with exercise equipment.

Peter had himself suffered a spinal cord injury and experienced the facilities and efforts of one of the Project Walk centres in the USA. Project Walk is a programme dedicated to improving the lives of individuals who have sustained paralysis after suffering a devastating spinal cord injury. The name was frowned upon by some in the UK who saw it as setting up individuals for disappointment by over-promising something that could usually not be delivered. Others saw this as a worthy goal to strive for, even if it was not achievable for all.

The effort within Project Walk is made through an intense exercise-based therapy programme and the aim is to facilitate as much recovery as possible for everyone. Peter noted that nothing seemed to be available like this in the UK and set out to do something about it. Before long, Standing Start moved to a local commercial unit and recruited its first therapist. Over time, it morphed into Neurokinex.

A growing number of centres with similar intent are now being created across the UK. These typically offer a mix of intensive exercise and technology-based programmes to private clients with a disability. Some offer packages such as therapy 'holiday' weeks and stress the importance of the available technology to what they do. The technology in the mix will vary a great deal and might be intended to reduce the need for manual intervention – for example, making it possible for an individual to carry out more repetitions of an exercise by providing some support to the effort required by the user or guiding the path of a movement.

The most important question here is obviously: do these facilities produce results? This is quite hard to answer in a general way because each client will have a different potential for improvement, different goals and expectations in mind and varying levels of motivation. The individual will ultimately decide on the value for money and whether there is a gap between what the facility promised and what it achieved.

The feedback I get is that some people get good results, and some don't. The problem in rehabilitation is that it is often hard to give a guarantee of a particular degree of recovery. In many walks of life, we know that if we take certain steps, we will get a particular result; it is not so simple for rehabilitation.

As some of these centres become more and more expensive and seem to promise more results, there is certainly a risk of disappointment. What I do know is that exercise-based therapy works. It is better to look at the principles of effective training and exercise from the world of strength and conditioning. After all, although disability brings its additional complications, some of the principles of exercise and training still hold for any human.

KEY POINT

Intensive exercise-based therapy programmes, similar to Project Walk in the USA, are popping up around the UK. The aim is to facilitate as much recovery as possible for everyone, but beware of those facilities making promises that seem too good to be true. That's what they probably are.

Training and exercise

Rehabilitation progress provoked by exercise will tend to have plateaus. Let's imagine that you have attended an intensive-therapy holiday to get you to the next level. You loved it and made some useful functional goals that met your expectations. It was expensive, but at least you got positive results. What happens now, though?

If you think about it for a moment, you will need to commit to some form of ongoing exercise or training practice to maintain anything you have gained. Otherwise, the benefits of that expensive week will almost certainly evaporate over time.

None of us, disabled or not, can expect to exercise occasionally and keep the strength and fitness we have gained for a lifetime. The 'use it or lose it' principle kicks in yet again – the body always adapts to the demands placed upon it. That is good news when the demand is created by regular exercise, but not so good when our body adapts to a sedentary lifestyle.

Let's distinguish between the terms 'exercise' and 'training' as they are often confused. Exercise is physical activity that is performed for the effect it has today. It is done for its own sake and may well involve doing the same activities at the same intensity day after day.

You could argue that this is what most people going to a gym do. There is nothing inherently wrong with this; in fact, exercise may be sufficient to reduce the risk of secondary complications following a spinal cord injury. The participant achieves a particular level of fitness, probably enjoys themselves in the process and may be content with that.

Training is different in that it is directed towards achieving a particular improved performance goal in the future. When athletes train, they must follow a systematic process that aims to stimulate the body to adapt over time. The specific nature of the process matters if the athlete is to achieve their desired results. Someone training for a marathon, for example, will not use the same process as a powerlifter.

You can train to gain cardiovascular fitness and strength, or skills in movement coordination and muscle size, but the specific nature of the training programme will always vary depending on the goals. If you have prospects for rehabilitation and functional gains, think of what you are doing as a training process rather than exercise. The busiest spot in most gyms is in front of the mirrors, but you may need to think less about exercising in front of the mirror if you want to make progress.

Coach, athlete and educator Eric Helms and his co-authors consider a hierarchy of parts of a training process (Helms, 2019). The authors describe this as a pyramid with the items of the most importance at the base supporting the others. In order of priority are:

1. Adherence

2. Volume, intensity and frequency

3. Progression

4. Exercise selection

5. Rest

6. Tempo

Spanning and supporting each of these components is the concept of 'periodisation'. We will get to this in a moment.

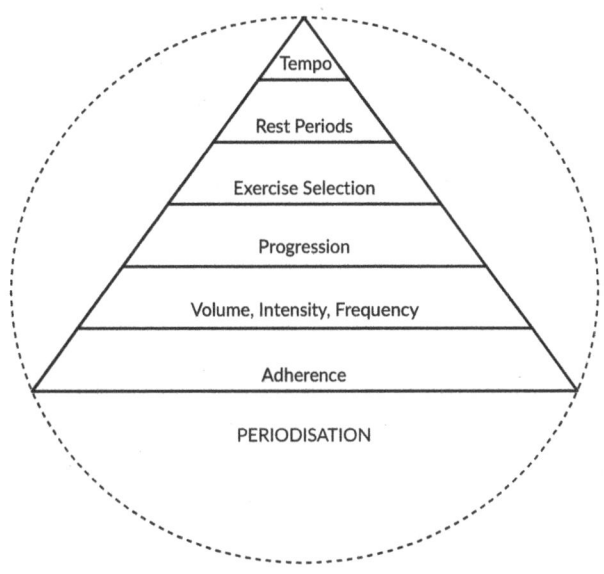

The training pyramid

If we think about what we have learned about neuroplasticity, the parameters we seem to have to influence are like those in the list and image above. In simple terms, periodisation is the intentional manipulation of training variables over time to achieve specific goals. Training for physical rehabilitation depends on tapping into the body's natural ability to respond and adapt to an applied stimulus. Remember the task specific, intensive and frequent approach to making gains in rehabilitation? Periodisation is how training should be structured to allow the body to adapt and grow fitter or stronger over time.

Before spending time thinking about the nuts and bolts of a training programme to recover function, we need to deal with the fundamental issue of adherence. This is the foundation of everything in training.

Basically, we humans are only likely to stick at something if certain conditions are met. There is no point designing a programme that we cannot commit to. The basic conditions are:

- **Is the training plan realistic?** You might have a particular functional improvement in mind, but you will need to have the time and resources to commit to the training otherwise you are not going to be successful. Is the training facility miles away and expensive to attend? If it is, the plan may not get off the ground.

- **Is it likely to be enjoyable?** Some people I know are hardcore and can focus on a distant abstract goal and keep going until they achieve it. This is typical of athletes and sports-oriented people who are comfortable with working hard towards achieving a goal even when the odds seem to be stacked against them, but most of us are not like that. We must work at finding the passion to keep going. A realistic appraisal of your ability to work towards a goal is important to how you can commit to a particular training plan. For example, do you work best in a one-to-one situation with a trainer, or would you thrive in a group environment?

- **Is the plan flexible?** As you are likely to need to work at improvement for the long term, there will be times when life gets in the way. No one wants to spend their life in therapy all the time, so does the plan allow for the unexpected? What happens if your energy levels are low one day?

Training for improvement typically uses the three qualities of volume, intensity and frequency, which to some extent are interrelated, to describe the variables. In strength and conditioning training, rules of thumb, increasingly backed by research, can guide you in how to set these variables to have different effects. For example, you might describe the training volume as the number of sets and repetitions of an exercise you carry out per week. Varying the intensity of effort used to carry out the volume of work is likely to produce different effects on the musculoskeletal and nervous system. Frequency relates to how often you carry out the prescribed volume of exercise.

In strength and conditioning training, to a certain extent, the volume of exercise has a dose-response relationship to strength and/or hypertrophy (muscle size gains), but this relationship is not linear. You'll eventually reach the point where your progress plateaus and even regresses as the volume of work increases. This is an individual characteristic and differs greatly between the novice trainee and the athlete, so it is hard to generalise; just be aware that there is no universal training programme or exercise you can adopt.

When it comes to training with a spinal cord injury, the principles of exercise still apply. It will be important to understand the application of adherence in each case and explore the variables of volume, intensity and frequency. You could refer to these three variables as the exercise dose, but unfortunately, you won't know beforehand how changing the dose might produce different effects.

All biological systems, including humans, adapt to the stimulus inherent in our environment. If we are sedentary, our body will apply its 'use it or lose it' mechanism to adapt to these circumstances. Equally, our body will adapt to the stimulus of a particular regime of exercise, and then ultimately progress will plateau.

In the figure below is a representation of what happens when humans train to achieve their physical potential. We could be talking about cardiovascular fitness or training for strength; the same pattern would apply.

The horizontal axis represents the timescale, for example in years of training, and the three curves represent the performance gained, the body's ability to adapt to the stimulus of exercise and the complexity of exercise the individual needs to provoke adaptation towards their physical potential. In the early days of training, the person is a beginner and rapidly gaining performance towards their potential. At this time, the complexity of training they need to provoke change is likely to be low and their ability to respond to exercise is high, but over time, to continue to make functional gains, they will need to change their exercise dose.

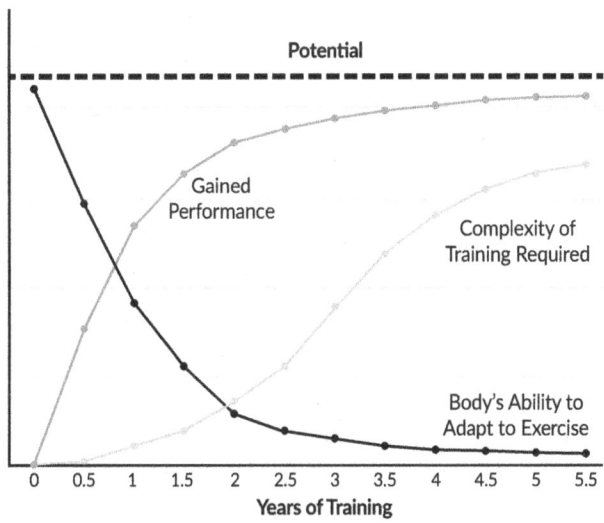

Training graph

For example, it might be necessary for them to change the volume, intensity or frequency of a certain exercise. The factors of exercise selection, speed of exercising and rest intervals between sessions are important in altering the stimulus that will force the body to respond, too.

Although this pattern relates to uninjured people training, the general principles surely apply for those with a disability. Some believe that to make gains as a disabled person, we must just keep going with the mantra that we need exercise to be specific, frequent and intensive, but it's not actually that simple. We might need to learn some lessons from strength and conditioning training. Almost every human can benefit from greater strength as well as cardiovascular fitness; in fact, when we are training for strength, we are also training our neurological system.

In strength and conditioning training, exercise selection is subject to the need to balance two contradictory things: specificity and variety. The best way of improving overall performance is to carry out a specific exercise repeatedly as this develops both skill and strength, but as the body adapts to the stimulus over time, it becomes necessary to add variety so that progress can continue. Variety of exercise provokes the body to carry on adapting.

Even people with ASIA A complete injuries can use FES cycling to pursue cardiovascular fitness and develop their limb muscle strength and joint ranges of motion. Periods of rest and recovery are also important in all physical training, so an effective exercise programme pays attention to both.

KEY POINT

There is no point in committing to an intensive-therapy week without recognising that training to achieve a functional goal is a continual journey. Most of us train or exercise to achieve a better quality of life, so we also need a balance between seeking fitness and getting on with life.

Nutrition following injury

I was listening to a radio debate where one party was saying eating too much red or processed meat increases our risk of bowel cancer, which definitely sounds like a bad thing. A second party pointed out that our risk of developing cancer because of eating meat is, in fact, small and it only makes a tiny difference to our overall risk. It's hard to get nutritional advice that isn't intentionally or unintentionally biased.

As a university academic, I would inform students that everything I was going to tell them was probably a lie – but at least, for now, a useful lie. This is because what we 'know' in many walks of life is based on what we might think of as the best evidence we have available at the time, but often we find that new evidence turns up that reveals a new and sometimes dramatically different understanding of how things work. That is certainly the case when it comes to nutrition.

A quick web search for nutritional guidelines following a spinal cord injury will reveal many sources of information and probably a good deal of consensus, but don't take such guidance as anything more than a best guess to follow for the time being. Nutritional guidance following a spinal cord injury is a complex and multifactorial challenge, so anything you read about this topic is – like my university lectures – no more than a useful lie. That's also true about exercise and nutritional guidance in general; we all need to approach the topic with a healthy dose of scepticism.

When we look at the topic of nutrition, it's like trying to see the whole of an elephant with a microscope: we will always have a limited view of the whole thing. The more we look at the details, the more complex we'll find it is.

What we know about eating well

It makes sense to consider what 'eating well' means for the general population first, and then look at the consequences that arise following a spinal cord injury. Good health depends on good nutrition; it's no secret that food directly affects how we look and feel and how our bodies work, so eating well logically seems to be the key to providing energy for life. It should boost our immune system, help us regulate our weight and keep all our body systems, including our brain, working in harmony to prolong our active lives. Experts tend to agree that every physiological process in our body is wholly dependent upon the nutrients in our diets and influenced by the less than nutritive substances we choose to consume.

Unfortunately, we still know little about exactly what eating well really means. Most of the information presented to us is based on some type of diet – I'm sure you will have seen a variety of fad diets come and go based on a particular paradigm. These fads are typically aimed at a common problem of losing weight, but they may not lead to optimal health.

Fitness is not about simply seeking to look better in the mirror, so nutritional excellence should not be based just on an ability to lose weight. It's no coincidence that these diets work for some people for a while, but then they disappear from public consciousness to be replaced by the next fad. Something is not right. It appears that in general, we humans tend to eat too much of the wrong foods at the wrong times. Too many of us are overweight and prone to metabolic disorders.

Researchers have looked back at our evolutionary history and to the emergence of homo sapiens around 200,000 years ago for clues to what nutrition we might really need. In evolutionary terms, our bodies have changed very little since that time, but the society in which we live has certainly not been stable. Some 99.99% of our genes were formed before the development of agriculture and shaped by the foods and selection pressures that were in the environments experienced by our ancestors. They faced uncertain food availability and knew nothing of the foods of modern commerce, which are often highly refined and processed.

It's reasonable to suggest that we have never evolved to adapt to the manufactured and highly processed foods that so often dominate our diets today. If we look around, we might feel that indeed we do eat too much of the wrong foods. Research suggests that our lifestyle and nutritional choices are interfering with our metabolism, which is ideally balancing two natural forces – autophagy and mechanistic target of rapamycin (mTOR) (Clement et al, 2019).

We can think of autophagy as a sort of cellular housekeeper responsible for burning fat reserves and cleansing the body of defective cells. mTOR, meanwhile, is a process of muscle building and fat storage. Detailed discussion of these forces is beyond the scope of this book, except to say that many diseases and our rate of ageing has been linked to dysregulation of mTOR.

Nutrition and stress

The world is certainly experiencing an ageing epidemic with a growing percentage of our population facing age-related diseases such as diabetes, heart disease, cancers and dementia. The root of the problem seems to be that we have a body that has not continued to evolve in step with the environment of stress humans must deal with today. Recent research suggests that the body's ageing has more to do with stress than our biological age and there is such a thing as beneficial stress (Hofmekler, 2017). It seems, though, there is a thin line between beneficial stress, which can extend life, and harmful stress, which will shorten life.

In popular culture, stress is seen as bad and to be avoided, but that might not be the best approach if we want to live long and healthy lives. We looked at stress in an earlier chapter from the point of view of our in-built stress-response system – the ANS. This system is optimised for short-term threats that we can literally fight or flee from. Unfortunately, we live in a modern world where our environment of stress can be sustained.

Let's examine stress in more detail from a nutrition viewpoint. In evolutionary terms, stressors were things such as lack of food, immediate danger to life, physical hardship or toxins. Our response to these stressors would include searching for food, fight or flight and detoxification. Stress millennia ago was only intermittent and usually not long lasting, but there is an important fact that we can't ignore. Stress today is very different from that faced by our ancestors and is often frequently experienced and long lasting. It's the energy bill we can't afford; the daily commute in busy traffic; the aggressive boss we can't avoid. The consequence of this is we get out of hormonal balance.

Hormesis

The impact of stress on biological systems has been a topic of interest for hundreds of years. The sixteenth-century Swiss physician, Paracelsus, described hormesis, which is based on the concept that a little bit of stress, applied the right way, can cause a biological system to adapt, and then become more resistant to a variety of stressful conditions. Paracelsus is reported to have said that, 'All things are poison and nothing is without poison; only the dose makes a thing not a poison' (Stringer and Rossiter, 2017). This is a case of the body naturally making stress work for us rather than against us. It sounds contrary to everything we may have thought was true.

A key issue is what constitutes a 'little bit of stress'. Exercise (a type of stress) can cause a beneficial adaption in our body. One consequence of this stress adaptation induced by hormesis is slower ageing and a corresponding delay in the onset of the chronic diseases and disabilities that tend to go along with ageing. Exercise can help to switch on autophagy, but if the amount of stress crosses a threshold, then we can be damaged.

Health experts such as Ori Hofmekler suggest that we are living in a world of anti-hormesis in which we generally have too much food of the wrong type that we eat at the wrong time (Hofmekler, 2017). As a result, we have too little exposure to the type of environmental stress that humanity evolved to deal with.

You have probably heard the expression 'What doesn't kill us will make us stronger', even if you don't believe it. Hofmekler points out that natural selection does work that way – in evolutionary terms, the underfed are selected for longevity and the overfed for ageing. Being underfed from time to time seems to switch on autophagy and turn off mTOR. Hofmekler describes the seven principles of stress, which are certainly thought provoking and contrary to what many of us may have believed. I encourage you to check out his views, which are challenging but fit with a great deal of what we know at present for nutritional health.

Anti-hormetic food

Anti-hormetic food ingredients are normal substances that, in effect, are toxic to the body. They are stress response inhibiting and are suspected to damage our ability to resist daily stressors and maintain good health. In this group are ingredients such as sugar, refined flour, artificial sweeteners, alcohol, monosodium glutamate and genetically modified organisms. These are associated with insulin resistance, obesity, diabetes, depression, premature ageing, inflammation and stress intolerance.

Let's take a quick look at three of these that are most important due to their frequency of use. Sugar is a commonly available substance that is strongly anti-hormetic because it has fast energy-releasing properties that can quickly inhibit the stress response. Taken in excess, sugar is toxic, but Hofmekler notes that added sugar is toxic even when consumed in amounts that are generally considered moderate. Whole foods that contain naturally occurring sugars such as fruit and root vegetables are, on the other hand, safe and viable.

Fructose is a component of sugar that naturally occurs in fruit, where it exists alongside co-factors that allow for its digestion and use by the body, but 'industrial' or refined fructose is more toxic than sugar itself. Avoid this as it is disruptive of your metabolism: it bypasses the insulin response and is challenging for organs that are insulin-dependent, such as the liver. Industrial fructose is commonly available in the forms of crystalline fructose and high fructose syrup, both derived mainly from corn. This refined fructose is found in many foods and drinks, including crackers, flavoured yoghurt, tomato sauce and salad dressing. Low-fat foods are often sweetened this way.

Artificial sweeteners were created as the 'calorie-free' alternatives to sugar and have been embraced by dieters and diabetics during recent years. These are not just the little pills you can pop into coffee and tea; these sweeteners are found in many products including diet drinks, low-carb and nutrition bars, and chocolates and sugar-free ice creams. A study reported in the journal *Nature* reveals that these substances can actually promote obesity and diabetes-related disorders more aggressively than sugar itself (Suez et al, 2014).

I have taken you to the edge of a deep rabbit hole of nutritional thinking and hopefully provoked your interest to challenge conventional ideas about nutrition. Now we need to get on to safer ground and consider the specific case of nutrition for spinal cord injury.

Nutrition and spinal cord injury

The resting metabolic rate of people with an injury is estimated to be 14–27% lower than that of their non-injured counterparts, largely due to reductions in fat-free mass and sympathetic nervous system activity (Buchholz et al, 2003). Most people lose some weight after injury as the body tries to self-repair from the stress imposed, so initially, the metabolic rate rises, but this is only temporary. Physical activity levels of people with an injury are generally lower than those of non-injured people, so weight gain becomes the obvious issue after a while.

In addition to this, some individuals post-injury can have substantial limitations to their effective independence, so caregivers play a large role in meal planning and diet adherence. Compared to the general population, people with spinal cord injuries are prone to two diet-related problems: heart disease and diabetes. For reasons that are not fully understood, blood chemistry becomes impaired: insulin tolerance is too high. In other words, the body produces more and more of the hormone insulin to transport energy to the body tissues. This is one of the known pathways to develop diabetes. Meanwhile, 'bad' cholesterol and triglycerides are too high, and 'good' cholesterol is too low.

In fact, little is known about the role of nutrition following a spinal cord injury and it is still unclear how it impacts body composition and the metabolic profile, so there are no clear universal guidelines for injured people to manage their metabolic profile. The common advice is basically what doctors say to everyone: moderate your lifestyle; don't eat so much; get some exercise; don't smoke; don't allow yourself to gain weight.

For some individuals with high-level injuries, it isn't just the type and quantity of food that's an issue; it's the way the food is presented. People who have problems swallowing must pay attention to the consistency and texture of foods, which should be soft and cut into small pieces that need minimal chewing. If food or drinks are too runny, some of the liquid can run into the airway to the lungs and cause coughing.

Bowel management is also directly related to diet. Since the muscular movements of the bowel are typically disrupted after spinal cord injury because of alterations to the central or peripheral nervous system, it's difficult for food to move through the intestinal system. A high-fibre diet and plenty of fluids are generally recommended. Sources of fibre include vegetables, fruits and nuts, and some people take supplements. High-fat foods should be avoided as they don't easily move through the body.

Pressure ulcers are common in individuals with high-level injuries, and if the worst should occur, healing can be compromised by their nutritional status. People with a pressure ulcer may have lower zinc, albumin and pre-albumin levels (Benton et al, 2019). Following a high-fibre diet can reduce the risk of poor healing rates.

KEY POINT

We are still pretty much in the dark as to what constitutes 'good' nutrition after a spinal cord injury. The best we can do is to follow the current guidelines, avoiding foods we know to be 'bad', such as sugar and refined flour, and making sure we take in plenty of fibre.

Summary

There is much to learn from looking at how strength and conditioning training works. This approach needs to be modified to suit the individual's exercise capability after a spinal cord injury, but the main lessons remain the same. Exercise is medicine and everyone can do something, but it's no good if it's just a one-occasion event. The body will only adapt to exercise that you take consistently, so you need to make sure it's something you can enjoy.

While high-tech ways of carrying out rehabilitation can appear attractive, they are not the only way of making progress. After all, the best form of exercise is that which you can continue to do. Simple methods allow everyone access, irrespective of financial resources or location.

Nutrition following a spinal cord injury is just as important as exercise, but it's an area where we need more research. Our understanding of nutrition is incomplete, but we can follow the best advice currently available for our individual circumstances. Certainly, avoiding substances that are known to challenge our metabolism makes sense.

Joe English's story

On 19 November 2017, Joseph English was involved in an accident when his brother Paul fell asleep at the wheel of his vehicle. The van veered off to the side of the road, hit a tree, flipped on to its side and crashed into the back of a parked car. As no airbags had gone off at the time of impact, Joe ended up with his head in the driver's footwell and his legs in the passenger's side. Surprisingly, he didn't have one visible injury to his body or face, but he had suffered a high-level spinal cord injury.

Joe was airlifted to Leeds General Hospital intensive care (his accident later appearing on the TV programme *999: Rescue Squad*). The doctors said he would not make it through the first twenty-four hours, but Joe surpassed all their expectations. After spending seven weeks in intensive care, he became strong enough to move to Sheffield Spinal Injury Unit where he spent eleven months.

Discharge was an extremely difficult time for him: adjusting to new ventilators and preparing himself and his care team for life at home, as well as dealing with the anxiety of being away from the hospital for the first time in twelve months. What if anything should go wrong? He was supported by a care agency to help with the clinical competencies and need for safety at home, but in the early days, Joe did struggle, including splitting up from his partner at the time.

After two years of difficult debate with the involved legal teams, he was awarded his first interim payment from a medico-legal claim. This afforded private physios, a psychologist, smart home technology and a dietician.

He and his team now know exactly how to look after his body clinically and have developed stretching programmes and pressure-relieving techniques while he's in his bed and wheelchair. This all helps to keep his skin and body healthy. With the help of a specialist dietician, he's lost over 2.5 stone and got down to a healthy weight.

Not everyone is lucky enough to be awarded an insurance claim, so Joe wants to pass his experience and knowledge on to help people in his position. Quad-Rebuild was founded by Joe in 2018 while he was spending his time in the spinal-injury unit (English, no date). He faced a difficult rehabilitation programme and recognised that thousands more people throughout the UK were in the same position. Many individuals were either waiting for discharge to a social care house or having to go into a care home because they could not afford to adapt their own home.

Lying in a hospital bed, day after day, feeling frustrated and helpless, he formed the idea of providing acute mentoring to support in-patients. Although Joe was still adjusting to his own life, he wanted to make a difference to others like him.

Joe's background was construction. He had set up his own business at the age of twenty and developed a strong reputation in the industry, so he now understood both the techniques of building and the needs of the disabled like himself. He has gone on to refine the key motives for his charity to 'Rebuilding lives, Rebuilding homes, Rebuilding your image and Rebuilding your future'.

Joe understands that to rehabilitate a person in all areas of their life, it is important to tailor a complete programme bespoke to their needs. Supporting an individual in the community is the final step to rebuilding their life.

You can read about Joe's project at www.quad-rebuild.co.uk.

SIX
Technology

As I make a living by offering technology for rehabilitation, you might expect this would be where I'd place the greatest emphasis. In fact, technology can allow us to do many things that would otherwise be impossible, but in my view it's just one ingredient for successful rehabilitation.

As with any tool, technology needs to be used with skilled direction and at the right time. Some technology is aimed at helping with restitution of function and some is fundamentally assistive and aimed at compensating for functional deficits. It is useful to grasp what you expect the technology to do for you and question the value of anything offered to you in your individual circumstances.

Inevitably, this chapter will be the fastest to date as new knowledge and products emerge. You may also find it more technical and challenging to read than earlier ones, so feel free to pick and choose the parts of most interest and treat the others as a reference you can come back to later if necessary.

Regaining or enhancing walking function

Do you want to walk again? According to some research literature, being able to walk again is often a priority among individuals with all levels of spinal cord injury, whatever their age (Ditunno et al, 2008). My experience is a little different from this suggestion; walking again is not generally number-one priority among my clients, whose point of view tends to change, dependant on the time since their injury, as they learn to accept that walking might never be possible for them. For example, people who have a high-level injury and are ventilated tend not to score walking as important compared with regaining more basic bodily functions. Paraplegics may rate walking as important more than those with cervical injuries – but only after bowel and bladder control and sexual function.

In the past, clinicians would be keen to tell most patients that walking would not be a possibility for them, but attitudes and beliefs tend to change as new evidence emerges. The recognition of the nervous system's ability to exhibit neuroplasticity has given rise to optimism about what might be possible, if not now, then in the future.

TECHNOLOGY

I have many clients who want to exercise and keep as fit as they can to take advantage of any new medical science advances that emerge in the future. The challenge is to understand that we all need hope and should not allow others to kill off this hope, but we still need to deal with the practical realities of what is possible today. The higher the level of complete injury, the less likely it is that walking will be possible due to the paralysis of the lower limbs.

To stand and move, humans must dynamically control the positions of multiple joints and limb segments. Walking is an inherently unstable activity, and we take each step in the presence of gravity, which imposes forces we must overcome to move. At some instances during walking, a particular joint must flex or extend, and at other times it will be stationary as the limb segments transmit the forces generated.

In health, we all walk without consciously having to think too much about it. We have an awareness of our limb positions (proprioception sense); it all just works. Our body-mind system deals largely unconsciously with how to orchestrate this complex activity at a high level.

Rehabilitation could be thought of as a process of recovering as much function as possible (restitution), followed perhaps by ultimately compensating for any function that we cannot recover. For many years, orthotic bracing has been the main approach to supporting the limbs paralysed by injury – we will consider orthotics shortly. In the past, we typically wouldn't expect to recover walking function naturally once we'd lost it, so if we wanted to walk, our best option would have been to use an orthosis with all the limitations that would bring. Recently, though, things have changed.

Beginning in the latter part of the twentieth century, several treadmill-based locomotor training approaches were developed with the ambitious goal of improving walking function in people with motor-incomplete injuries. These approaches relied on the concept of central pattern generators, which are specialised systems of cells located in the spinal cord that provide the basic step rhythms for walking (Grillner et al, 1998). You could think of these pattern generators as the high-level nervous system programmes that allow walking to be a behaviour we don't normally have to think too much about. They are literally hardwired in the body for us to use.

Research had demonstrated that animals with completely severed spinal cords could walk proficiently on a treadmill with partial body weight support (Forssberg, 1980a and 1980b). The theory behind this research is that the movement of the legs by the treadmill activates sensory afferents in the limbs that in turn switch on the spinal central pattern generators. In other words, signals generated in the limbs flow towards the central nervous system and turn on the pattern generators. The result of this training is rhythmic stepping, timed to the movement of the treadmill.

The change in excitability of the specific neural circuits engaged in the training activity is a necessary component of neuroplasticity. The question then

TECHNOLOGY

arises: can we enhance the effect by using some additional form of stimuli?

Evidence suggests that several non-invasive but clinically accessible forms of stimulus energy, such as electrical, magnetic and vibration, may augment the effects of treadmill training (Iyer et al, 2003). In essence, stimulation can activate the same neural circuits that are activated by the treadmill training. When used in combination with such training, it has the potential to promote neuroplasticity beyond that achieved by practice or training alone.

Research has suggested that stimulation can serve as a mechanism to prime the nervous system (Iyer et al, 2003), thereby increasing its receptiveness and responsiveness to other forms of repetitive training. Indeed, several studies have shown that stimuli that increase neural excitability will also increase responsiveness to motor training. As an example, FES has been used for decades as an adjunct to locomotor training in people with spinal cord injury (Barbeau et al, 2002).

As FES activates both sensory and motor neural elements, from the perspective of maximising the contribution of spinal circuits, it may be of value to augment afferent input beyond that supplied by the moving treadmill alone. Electrical stimulation has been incorporated into locomotor training with the goal of exciting the flexor reflex afferents, which are thought to be involved with the spinal-locomotor pattern-generating circuitry. Combining functional electrical stimulation-evoked afferent input with the input supplied by the moving treadmill should theoretically provide optimal drive to the spinal-locomotor centres and positive outcomes in terms of walking speed and distance, as well as improved limb coordination (Field-Fote and Tepavac, 2002).

What about vibration as the stimulus? In neurologically healthy individuals, localised vibration to the leg muscles has been shown to influence locomotor activity (Ivanenko et al, 2000). It has been proposed that this effect is due to activation of spinal central pattern generator mechanisms. A theory is that vibration excites spinal central pattern generator circuits that underlie the generation of locomotor output contributing to walking function.

In contrast to localised muscle vibration, whole-body vibration (WBV) represents a generalised form that seems to have more widespread effects. This may represent a viable approach to priming the spinal circuits to increase responsiveness to locomotor training. Based on this evidence for the value of WBV in promoting improved locomotion, a study of participants with chronic motor-incomplete injury investigated the effect of a twelve-session WBV intervention on walking function (Ness and Field-Fote, 2009). All subjects had limited walking function and used a wheelchair as their primary means of moving around. Results indicated that the WBV intervention was associated with a significant increase in walking speed for this subject population (Musselman, 2007).

Peripheral nerve stimulation, muscle vibration and WBV all target spinal mechanisms that contribute to lower extremity motor control and walking function. Transcutaneous spinal cord stimulation and transcutaneous spinal direct current stimulation represent emerging approaches that target spinal cord circuitry more directly. We will look at transcutaneous spinal cord stimulation in a later section.

KEY POINT

The recognition of the nervous system's ability to exhibit neuroplasticity has given rise to optimism about what might be possible either now or in the future.

Orthotic bracing

An orthosis is a structure that is added to the body to control one or more limb segments or joint motions and redirect forces for therapeutic effect. If that sounds a bit vague, it is because orthotics is a broad topic. An orthosis may be applied to many body parts, including the upper limbs, the legs, the extremities or the neck and trunk. It may be designed to prevent or correct deformity or to provide support for an activity such as walking in cases of paralysis.

The principle of putting force to work for therapeutic purpose is often associated with the so-called Tree of Andry.

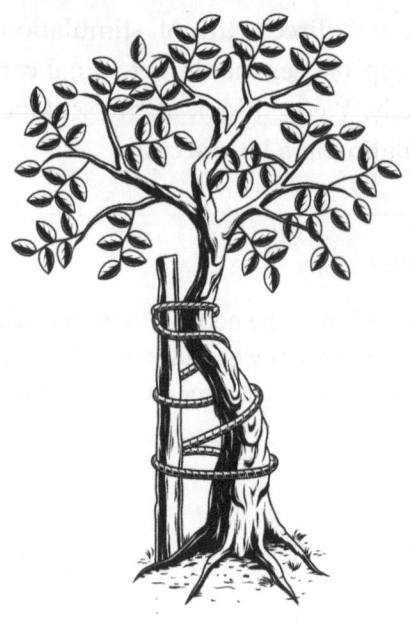

Tree of Andry

Nicholas Andry holds an important place in the history of medicine as it was he who first used the word 'orthopaedics' in a book published in 1741 (Kohler, 2010). Within the text, he illustrated the crooked tree which has become the symbol for many orthopaedic organisations around the world and can also be a metaphor for orthotics. Although many related agencies have taken to modifying or customising the tree, the essential design remains the same.

TECHNOLOGY

Orthoses have been made for hundreds if not thousands of years to support body parts affected by disease or trauma. In past times, these products may have been made from leather or steel and shaped by craftsmen to fit the individual's body as intimately as possible. These craftsmen probably knew little about anatomy and physiology, so orthoses would often have been of limited effectiveness due to their weight. They may also have been perceived as ugly contraptions, a necessary evil.

More recently, custom orthoses have been fashioned from lightweight mouldable plastic materials such as polypropylene combined with steel joints when necessary.

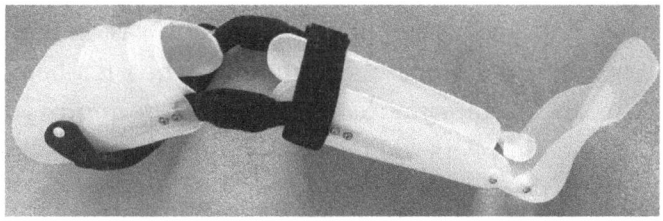

An example of a custom polypropylene orthosis that spans the whole leg and is jointed at the knee and ankle

To ensure an intimate contact with the tissue, the body of the orthosis would often be formed from a plaster model made directly from the person's body part. This plaster model would be modified during the manufacturing process to allow the finished orthosis to be more effective in how it interfaced with the body: an orthosis needs to apply force to the body that it interacts with in an intimate way without those forces damaging potentially insensitive tissue.

Today, orthotics is a profession in which practitioners are well-educated clinicians with a good understanding of the mechanics of materials, the anatomy and the biomechanics of the human body. In the UK, Prosthetics (limb replacement) and Orthotics is a regulated allied health profession and those in practice have to follow a prescribed training course of instruction that includes theoretical and practical elements.

Passive orthotic devices today can take advantage of materials such as carbon fibre composites that allow a lightweight, strong and cosmetic appearance. Reduction in weight and an intimate fit to the body are important aspects of a passive orthosis as these reduce the additional encumbrance when it's being worn, and its appearance is also likely to be improved.

Some suppliers are experimenting with 3D scanning and printing technology. This has been in development since the 1980s as a prototyping technology, but in more recent times it has increasingly offered the capability to allow direct manufacture of orthoses. While this approach offers many advantages for trying out ideas, it still generally requires a high capital cost if direct manufacture is the aim.

As we've learned, an orthosis is added to the body to fix or control a segment or joint motion due to a functional deficit. It must do this despite the forces generated by activity. Where a spinal cord injury results in lower-limb paralysis, for example, the muscles surrounding the joints can no longer generate the power to move the limbs or even maintain the limb positions in passive standing. In some cases, contractures can develop in the ankles or hands and arms, and an orthosis might be used to manage these contractures.

In relation to the lower limbs, depending on the extent of the paralysis, an orthosis could be created for the ankle and foot (AFO), to span the knee, ankle and foot (KAFO) or even the hip, knee, ankle and foot (HKAFO). The orthosis, when positioned on the affected limb, acts to stabilise the joints, preventing unwanted flexion or extension. In many cases, this can allow the person to stand or even walk with the aid of forearm crutches or a rollator.

When the spinal cord injury is incomplete and/or at a low level on the spine, meaning the foot and ankles and at most the knee joints require support, orthotic devices might be a good choice to allow some standing and mobility. In this case, the additional encumbrance introduced by adding the orthosis to the body may be low enough that the user will feel they gain more than they lose in terms of function. If the user finds that the effort of walking with a passive orthosis is too high compared with the convenience of using a wheelchair, it's likely they will not use the orthosis.

Orthoses should be prescribed and created by registered orthotic professionals, who may work for the NHS (in the UK), provide services privately or be employees of private companies that act as contractors to the NHS. For best results, especially to ensure insensitive skin is protected, orthotics should be custom made. Lightweight materials are most likely to result in the lowest encumbrance to use.

Some orthosis designs have jointed structures, allowing some controlled movement. For example, KAFO designs can ensure the knee is locked and stable during the stance phase of walking, yet free to move during the swing phase of gait. These devices may have mechanical joints or even electromechanical joints that aim to improve usability.

In my early career in Canada, I worked with many children with spina bifida (a form of spinal cord defect present at birth). The children with a sacral or lumbar level injury could often use an AFO or a KAFO when they were small, but invariably, they would choose to abandon their orthoses as they got older and bigger as the effort of walking with these passive structures became too much for them. Some clever innovations aimed to overcome this mechanical challenge, but even with lightweight materials, what these devices needed was an additional source of power. An orthosis that adds power to the body can potentially compensate for what the body has lost.

KEY POINT

Orthoses may look like simple structures, but they need to be carefully prescribed and manufactured for best effect. They are widely used for musculoskeletal injuries, but when they're used with spinal cord injuries, we must take extra care to protect insensitive skin from pressure ulcers.

Exoskeletons

Robotics and exoskeletons are eye-catching developments that have great potential. Orthotic devices have been used for generations to passively control and stabilise the legs, but unfortunately, the effort involved in ambulation has often been too much for many users, particularly when their spinal cord injury affected the trunk, thigh and shank muscles.

For many years, research has been developing soldier enhancement systems, particularly as part of the remit of the Defense Advanced Research Projects Agency in the USA. Infantry soldiers typically must carry loads greater than their body weight over long distances in difficult terrain, so technology that could support them to do this could prevent injury and extend load carrying ability.

By the year 2000, the first commercial exoskeletons were emerging, and it seems that new developers are continuing to appear all the time. According to the website www.exoskeletonreport.com, there are currently (in 2022) 118 exoskeleton developers, mostly located in Asia, Europe and North America. The exoskeleton industry is dominated by new start-ups, complemented by some well-established companies that have taken an interest in the technology.

The time between 2016 and 2017 had the highest number of new company creations. Not all of these companies focus on the medical market, though. A similar percentage focus on industrial applications; for example, to reduce workplace injuries in situations such as construction or vehicle manufacture where workers are typically having to move high loads or are subject to repetitive activities which can result in injury to the back or hands.

One of today's problems is that exoskeletons for medical applications have been subject to a lot of hype, which has led to unrealistic expectations. Science-fiction, such as the *Iron Man* movies, has excited lots of people in relation to exoskeleton technology, but we need a more measured conversation on what this technology can and can't do at this time. Taking on board completely unrealistic expectations, people can easily become disillusioned by the present reality of exoskeleton technology.

The arrival of the first powered lower-limb exoskeleton was greeted with some excitement by the rehabilitation community. Not everyone was a fan, though. A spinal-injury consultant and friend of mine described the early exoskeleton systems offered to clients as 'Expensive toys – little better than mobile standing frames'.

In one sense, he was right. The first products on the market were not necessarily acting to restore function beyond what was possible with a standing frame; they were purely assistive devices. The user could initiate movement, and then the design would take

TECHNOLOGY

over, electric motors within the structure providing the necessary power to stabilise and move the lower limbs. My friend understood that the novelty of being able to stand and move would probably wear off for the user, who could achieve the same clinical value more simply and cheaply by a regular regime of passive standing.

There is no doubt that the cost of these products has placed them outside of the price range of the majority of those who could use them. In the UK, users of the Indego Personal Exoskeleton have all so far successfully pursued a medico-legal case, but there are different drivers for adoption of the technology in different countries. For example, in the USA, qualifying injured veterans of the armed forces can be provided with an exoskeleton without charge to them. No such initiatives exist in the UK at the time of writing.

Where there is some potential for functional improvement (ie with an incomplete spinal cord injury), only some of the current exoskeletons can provide a truly restorative function. The buyer needs to be aware of this and make sure that a producer's claims are really justified as the restorative possibilities do vary significantly from device to device. If the user has a complete injury and no potential to recover function, an exoskeleton will have to provide all of the propulsive power as well as the structural stability to support the limbs. It will be acting purely as an assistive product, compensating totally for the lost function.

We are starting to see the emergence of wearable textile-based exoskeletons. These softer, more compliant structures are not likely to be helpful for a complete spinal cord injury as they cannot generate the necessary mechanical forces to stabilise the limbs, but they could be beneficial for some neurological conditions such as multiple sclerosis or post stroke.

The difference between a restorative and assistive exoskeleton was brought home to me following a discussion with Claire Lomas, whose case is included in an earlier chapter. Claire came to public fame when she walked the London Marathon using an exoskeleton to raise funds for spinal research. She had been in touch with me over the years as an enthusiastic daily user of my business's FES cycling system, which meant Claire has well-developed leg muscles. When spending time in her exoskeleton during the days of the London Marathon walk (it took her seventeen days), she noticed that her leg muscles diminished in size. Far from being restorative, the exoskeleton had contributed to loss of muscle bulk in her legs. Of course, the general benefits of standing and loading her leg bones would still be present, but these she could have got just as easily by using a standing frame.

An exoskeleton with restorative abilities will either have sensors and software intelligence to adjust the level of power assistance provided to the user automatically or allow real-time therapist intervention to fine tune the amount of support. This is all about providing a training effect to the user and ensuring that the exoskeleton motors are not just doing all the work. Some of the current exoskeletons can be purchased with built-in FES to stimulate the leg muscles in sync with the limb movements, which will also enhance the restorative function.

The present generation of exoskeletons can offer benefits not possible with passive orthotic devices, but currently this is at a relatively high cost. Each potential user will place a different emotional and practical value on the ability to stand and move in their home environment. As the calculation of benefit is an emotive one, purchasing an exoskeleton deserves careful consideration.

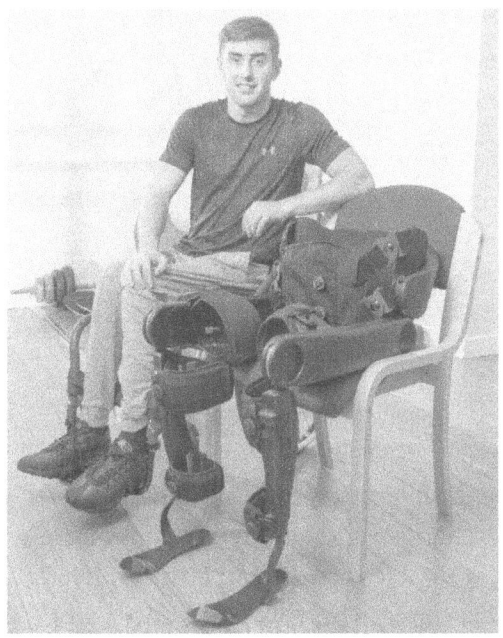

The Indego Personal Exoskeleton

It is certainly a good idea to try all of the exoskeleton systems that are available if you can. Remember too that you will likely take a bit of time to become proficient in using an exoskeleton. It's like learning to walk all over again as you will need to stand up, initiate walking, and then stop once more.

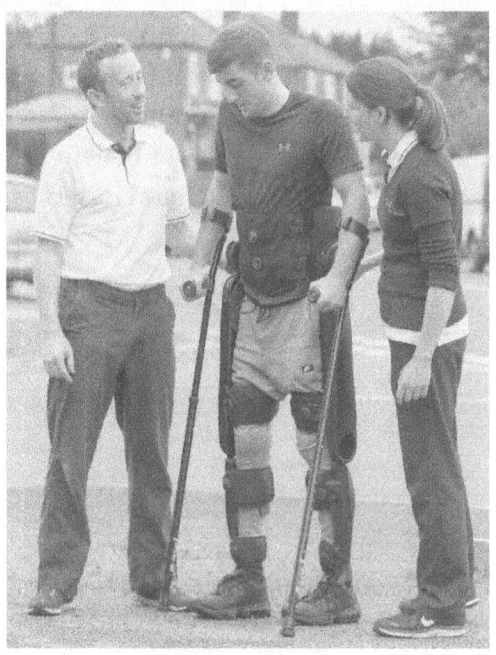

Training to use an Indego Exoskeleton

Just like humanity went through a digital revolution that changed the way we communicate with one another, wearable robotics can bring a physical revolution which changes how we think about work, therapy, disabilities, neurological conditions and even what it means to get old. One direction manufacturers are contemplating is to produce powered components to incorporate into more conventional orthotic products. This approach might bring the cost down while catering for the absence of power with conventional orthotics.

KEY POINT

When you're considering the purchase of an exoskeleton, ask yourself a few questions. Why would you want to purchase an exoskeleton in particular? What alternatives are there? What would you like to think, feel and do as a result? Is this purchase realistic based on guidance from your clinical advisors? What is the lifetime of this product?

Electrical stimulation

Various forms of electrical stimulation can be effective and safe for a wide variety of applications, but clinicians are not always in tune with what is possible. Let's start by looking back at the history of electrical stimulation, and then explore some modern-day applications.

In 1871, French physician Guillaume Duchenne was using electrical stimulation – *électrisation localisée* – to stimulate leg muscles to produce standing in paraplegic patients. I wasn't around in 1871, but about 100 years later I was introduced to using electrical stimulation to assist with drop foot following stroke.

The equipment wasn't as slick as that available today, but the advantages of this approach were clear.

In Canada in the 1970s, we were also using forms of electrical stimulation to correct idiopathic scoliosis in growing adolescents, with both surface and implanted electrodes, and to prevent the development of foot and ankle contractures in children with cerebral palsy. In the late 1970s and throughout the 1980s, though, it seemed to me that electrical stimulation had gone out of fashion. Maybe it was I who had gone out of fashion and wasn't tuned in to the trends.

The fact is that there may be more than one way of achieving a result and ways of doing things are influenced by the authority and relative status of any professions involved. For example, the therapists I worked with in the 1970s complained that the orthopaedic surgeons were quick to advocate surgery for tendon-Achilles lengthening for children with cerebral palsy rather than more conservative passive stretching approaches. The surgeons believed that if therapists could operate, they would be doing exactly the same, and their conservative methods would be forgotten.

When someone advocates a particular type of therapy, surgery or whatever, be aware that there may be other approaches that this person is not familiar with. While clinicians may focus on the availability of evidence to support an activity, it is rare to disconnect a technique from the knowledge and skills needed to apply it.

TECHNOLOGY

For example, Surgeon A publishes the results of a series of surgical cases with a new procedure. Other surgeons around the world copy the procedure. Some visit and work directly with Surgeon A and capture the subtleties not easy to describe in a text; some just read about the procedure and come up with their own interpretation, which is ultimately a failure. They then blame Surgeon A for the failures. Skill and experience count when it comes to weighing up the effectiveness of an approach.

For more than 200 years, we have known that electricity applied to the body can cause contraction of muscle. Generalising, we can say that the delivery of energy (in this case a form of electric current) to muscle tissues can bring about physiological changes in the tissues (often via nerve stimulation), thereby achieving therapeutic benefit. We could call this 'electrotherapy'.

The critical issue is how to set a machine in such a way as to stimulate the target nerves as effectively and efficiently as possible. Stimulation of sensory nerves can achieve a sensory outcome; similarly, stimulation of motor nerves will bring about a limb movement or motor effect. It is not possible to only stimulate one type of nerve or another, but it is possible to primarily influence a particular nerve type by setting appropriate parameters on the stimulation device. Some electrotherapy equipment in this area is specific and dedicated to a particular task while some offers many different stimulation modes and a selection can be made, typically from a menu system.

One of the confusing things about electrotherapy can be the terminology to describe different stimulation modes. Here are a few:

- NMES – neuromuscular electrical stimulation
- EMG-NMES – electromyography-triggered neuromuscular electrical stimulation
- EMS – electrical myostimulation
- FES – functional electrical stimulation
- TENS – transcutaneous electrical nerve stimulation
- cNMES – cyclic neuromuscular electrical stimulation
- IFT – interferential therapy
- Russian stimulation
- Diadynamic therapy

I could easily continue this list, but at present, there isn't a universally agreed classification system that applies to all known modalities and avoids ambiguities. For example, TENS is commonly thought of as sensory nerve stimulation used primarily for pain relief, but most other forms of stimulation are, strictly speaking, transcutaneous too because they involve the use of gelled surface electrodes. I am going to neatly sidestep this issue so as not to add to the confusion, using the term electrotherapy as the broad umbrella

TECHNOLOGY

and FES to describe applications where functional movement is the objective in rehabilitation.

Over the last fifty years our understanding has improved, and with it the technology to make FES one of the most powerful and flexible tools we have for rehabilitation. Despite its long pedigree, electrical stimulation is not well understood in its various forms or applied widely enough for therapeutic purposes. Of course, applying electricity to the body has to be done with knowledge of what is safe and effective.

I first worked with FES in the 1970s which is, by anyone's standards, a long time ago now. The technology available in those days was not so easy to use compared with the systems we have today. Many technologies seem to come in and out of fashion for a variety of reasons, but with FES, the growth in popularity is in part due to the increased sophistication made possible by developments in semiconductor and microprocessor technology. Modern systems offer fine control of the stimulation and as a result produce a more predictable result.

Whatever era we are in, the fundamental questions of interest remain the same:

- What can FES do that is worth the trouble?
- How does FES work?
- Is it safe to use? Will it damage healthy nerves and muscles?

- Can the central nervous system or a lower motor-neuron system be retrained or reorganised through FES?
- How can we design FES systems for maximum benefit?

We will now touch on some of these questions.

It was just prior to 1800 that Italian physician Luigi Galvani discovered that electricity applied to the sciatic nerve of a frog would produce a contraction of the frog's leg. This and the controversy between Galvani and a scientist called Alessandro Volta laid the foundations for FES.

Volta, a professor of experimental physics, was among the first to repeat Galvani's experiments. Initially, he embraced the idea of 'animal electricity', but Volta came to believe that the contractions depended on the metal cable Galvani had used to connect the nerves and muscles in his experiments. Galvani believed that the animal electricity came from the muscle in the frog's pelvis. Volta, in opposition, reasoned that the animal electricity was a physical phenomenon caused by rubbing the frog's skin and not a metallic electricity at all.

Volta's intuition was correct. In fact, every cell has an electrochemical potential. Biological electricity has the same chemical underpinnings as the current between electrochemical cells, so can be duplicated outside the body.

Volta essentially objected to Galvani's conclusions about 'animal electric fluid', but the two scientists disagreed respectfully and Volta coined the term 'Galvanism' for a direct current of electricity produced by chemical action. Owing to an argument between the two regarding the cause of the electricity, Volta built the first battery to specifically disprove his associate's theory, which became known as a voltaic pile.

During my PhD training, I was lucky enough to be able to study anatomy and dissection at the Glasgow University Anatomy Theatre. This place has a feel of history about it, so let me tell you a true story from the past (Ure, 1819).

The inside of the Glasgow University Anatomy Theatre was crowded. After all, it wasn't every day that anatomists worked on a fresh corpse in full public view. Five minutes before Matthew Clydesdale's corpse was brought from the gallows, Dr Andrew Ure charged his galvanic battery. A series of experiments were then carried out on the recently hanged body.

The final experiment involved the current being turned on. As soon as this happened, Clydesdale raised his hand and pointed to the people in the audience. Several spectators fled, terrified, from the arena and one fainted (Pattison, 1986).

In the nineteenth century, there was significant interest in electrotherapy. An electric bath was a medical treatment in which high-voltage apparatus electrified patients by causing a charge to build up on their bodies. In the USA, this process was known as Franklinization after Benjamin Franklin, as it became widely known when Franklin described it, but after that it was mostly practised by quacks.

Golding Bird brought it into the mainstream in the UK at Guy's Hospital in the mid-nineteenth century, but the approach fell into disuse in the early twentieth century.

FES is a therapy method where nerves are stimulated through the skin with precisely controlled electrical energy to cause a functionally useful muscular contraction. To understand how FES works, let's first look briefly at how muscles work normally.

Each skeletal muscle has a nerve architecture of thousands of fibres that generate force when they contract. A group of fibres is connected ultimately to the brain through a nerve cell called a motor neuron. This group of fibres and its motor neuron is referred to as a motor unit.

An individual muscle fibre either contracts or it doesn't; there is no middle ground. In essence, the nervous system tells the muscle to contract by the energy signal that flows along the nerve. Once this energy reaches a high enough level, muscle fibres are 'turned on' and contract.

How does a muscle manage to control the force it exerts? This is done by the nervous system varying the firing frequency at which the energy signal flows to the motor units. Firing the fibres with an increased frequency will increase the force generated and the power output. When firing is synchronised across many motor units, again, the force generated is increased. Normally, motor units take turns in firing to produce a controlled and smooth movement and

TECHNOLOGY

only a small percentage of the motor units available are recruited at any one time.

These motor units supply muscle fibres, sometimes a few and sometimes many dependant on the specific muscle. High-force postural muscles have many muscle fibres and low-force precise control muscles contain relatively few muscle fibres. Motor-unit recruitment, firing frequency and synchronisation are referred to as intramuscular coordination.

A spinal cord injury disrupts or disallows the energy signal that would normally enable this whole process to work. FES can be used in a relatively crude way to produce the energy signal that the nervous system can no longer deliver to the muscles. When in good health, the nervous system can skilfully recruit and orchestrate the many muscle contractions necessary to perform an everyday movement. No FES system exists that can replace this; the best we can do is to encourage functionally useful contractions of individual or groups of muscles.

A detailed description of FES is beyond the scope of this book, but I can give a brief outline of how it works in practice. The basic idea is that we have to replace the energy signal which would normally propagate along the nerves supplying each muscle. With FES, this energy is generated as an external electrical source and introduced to the body via either implanted or surface electrodes.

If we consider the surface electrode case, the electrical energy applied to the skin must penetrate the layers of dermal tissue and impact upon the local intact nerve structure. If the energy is sufficient, then muscle fibre recruitment takes place and the muscle contracts. Each nerve has a particular threshold of energy required to trigger an action potential, and activation and muscle contractions take place when the stimulation intensity is high enough.

In commonly available FES units, the electrical energy will consist of a bipolar rectangular pulse train. Typically, the frequency, pulse width and current levels of the pulse train will be adjustable. These three parameters will control the intensity of the muscle contraction, but each parameter may have a different effect.

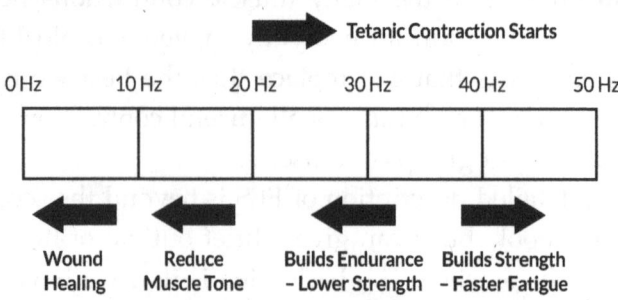

Effect of stimulation frequency on muscle

For example, increasing the frequency to 50 Hz will tend to generate great strength of muscle contraction, but lead to faster fatigue than a frequency of 30 Hz. Stimulators will typically offer ranges of adjustment from 5 to 50 Hz for frequency, a maximum pulse width of 500 microseconds and a maximum current level of 130 mA.

With FES cycling, which we review in the next section, we are looking for a training effect, so we will have to think about which muscles we need to train and what outcomes we want because this influences the choice of stimulation parameters. Electrical stimulation can produce the necessary muscle contractions to pedal a bike, but the muscles need to produce these contractions at the right time. The software and hardware used in FES cycling is designed to precisely control when particular muscles are stimulated.

KEY POINT

Biological electricity has the same chemical underpinnings as the current between electrochemical cells, so can be duplicated outside the body.

FES cycling

When we looked at Christopher Reeve's case, you might have noted that he used an FES cycling system as part of his intensive rehabilitation and fitness training. This is technology my business has worked with for many years now and it's used by hundreds of people in homes across the UK as well as hospitals and private therapy practices. It has proved to be a safe and efficient way for some people with a spinal cord injury to exercise.

In this section, we will look at the background to this technology and what it offers to users. FES cycling programmes are designed to synchronise the stimulation delivered to the major muscles with the movement of the bike's pedals. The quadriceps, hamstrings and other muscle groups involved in a stimulation programme are effectively turned on and off at the necessary times during each revolution. This means that a user with paralysed limbs can still exercise these limbs actively against resistance.

The stimulator and the bike communicate with each other during an exercise session, passing data back and forward. The stimulator always needs the position of the pedals so that it knows which muscles should be active at any instant. As the pedal speed increases, the software will automatically adjust the stimulation to suit. Of course, the stimulator software is watching for error situations which might indicate a problem, such as an electrode becoming detached or when the pedals stop moving suddenly due to a leg spasm.

In 2006, David Allan, at that time clinical director of the Scottish National Spinal Injuries Unit, introduced me to the German company HASOMED GmbH. HASOMED, the spinal unit and Glasgow University had been one of the major UK research groups looking at FES cycling and the three organisations were now wanting to see their research brought into practice.

TECHNOLOGY

In the early 1980s, research established that people with a spinal cord injury, including patients with a clinically complete lesion, are often able to propel a cycle by means of controlled sequential electrical stimulation of the large leg muscles (Petrofsky, 1984). In effect, the user's paralysed muscles can be made to contract sufficiently strongly and with controlled timing to pedal a bike. Typically, a motorised bike is integrated with a multichannel FES unit. In the image, a MOTOmed Loop LA is shown with the integrated eight-channel FES unit from HASOMED GmbH.

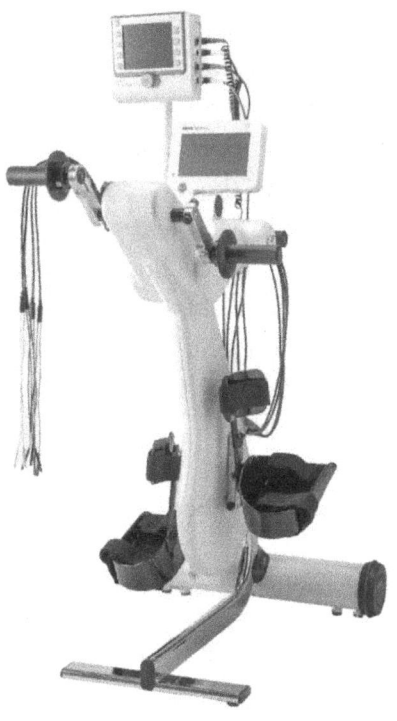

RehaMove based on Loop LA

The stimulation intensity can be automatically adjusted with the aim of encouraging an increase in cycling effort within safe limits. By this means, the user is able to cycle against resistance that can be increased as they get stronger. Although the motorised bike could move the legs passively (which has some benefit), the health benefits are much stronger if the exercise is active via the muscle stimulation.

FES cycling has typically utilised surface stimulation technology, where adhesive electrodes are attached to the surface of the skin over appropriate muscle motor points on the main limb segments. Typically, these electrodes are at least placed on the quadriceps and hamstrings, but the gluteal, tibialis anterior and gastrocnemius muscles may also be used. Some bikes support upper-limb applications; these typically involve the anterior and posterior deltoid, triceps and bicep muscles.

The feasibility of FES cycling as an effective exercise option has led to a large number of research studies to examine possible therapeutic and medical benefits which may help to reduce the general and wide-ranging secondary complications that often accompany a spinal cord injury. One review summarises the key potential benefits (Janssen et al, 1998):

- Improved muscle size and strength
- Increased range of joint motion
- Improved cardiopulmonary fitness and peripheral circulation

- Preservation of bone density
- Improved cosmesis
- Likely to reduce the impact of troublesome spasticity in the leg muscles

Like all training interventions, a lot depends on how this technology is used in practice. Certainly, one of the issues that worried me when I first started to work with FES cycling was whether people would actually use it. After all, not everybody who has a gym membership commits to regular attendance.

When we discussed strength and conditioning training, we looked at the importance of adherence. The best exercise programme is the one we can commit to. I was aware in the early days that if people did not use FES cycling products, then all the research and development effort would have been wasted. The benefits from FES cycling, just as with any type of exercise, only last if the person is using the system.

In a cycle training intervention report, ten complete-lesion subjects (with a level from C6–T4) completed an average of 2.3 half-hour cycling sessions per week over the course of one year (Mohr et al, 1997). The outcomes of this study included a significant (almost 20%) increase in peak oxygen uptake and a 10% increase in bone density measured in the proximal tibia using dual energy absorptiometry (DEXA scanning) (Mohr et al, 1997). It is notable that despite the rapid muscle loss that can occur following paralysis, a programme of FES cycling exercise may result in at least partial restoration of the depleted slow-oxidative muscle fibre population and re-capillarisation.

These days, FES cycling systems are often provided to spinal cord injured people as part of a medico-legal case. The evidence of value is strong for spinal cord injury and these systems represent one of the few ways that people with a complete injury can actively exercise their legs. A review of the literature confirms that current evidence indicates FES cycling exercise improves lower-body muscle health of adults with a spinal cord injury and may increase power output and aerobic fitness (van der Scheer et al, 2021).

Anyone thinking of using FES cycling should check for contraindications which might mean it is not safe for them to use the stimulation. Suppliers will typically offer a demonstration. As with any technology, there are both indications and contraindications for the benefits of FES cycling. People with a so-called denervation injury will not be able to use this system and we will discuss this next.

KEY POINT

FES cycling is a well-researched and safe method of exercising legs or other paralysed muscles with great health benefits. It is used by hundreds of people at home, but the muscles must be innervated for this to work.

TECHNOLOGY

Electrical stimulation of denervated muscle

FES cycling has become a well-evidenced and widely adopted modality for preserving long-term health in spinal cord injury, but not everyone will be able to use this system effectively. The type of muscle stimulation used by these bikes relies on an intact nerve structure within the leg muscles. In other words, the so-called lower motor neurons must be intact for the FES cycling system to produce effective muscle contractions. The energy signal depends on these motor neurons to initiate a muscle contraction, but injuries to the spinal cord below T10 or damage to a peripheral nerve may result in what is called denervation of the leg muscles.

The fundamental problem with denervated muscles is that the nerves degrade and cannot be used to trigger a contraction. Once this type of injury occurs, both the nerve and the muscle structure change over time. This results in a flaccid type of paralysis where the legs may become extremely wasted in appearance and especially prone to secondary problems. Denervated muscles can only be made to contract when muscle fibres are stimulated directly by relatively broad pulses with much greater levels of energy (millisecond) than the microsecond-wide pulses typically seen with FES. Sometimes much higher levels of current are necessary, too.

The problem with denervation is that skeletal muscle changes its structure in the absence of innervation and wastes away over time, leading finally to a state in which the functioning muscle tissue is largely replaced by fibrous connective tissue and fat, along with a scattering of extremely damaged muscle fibres. These muscle fibres are almost unrecognisable at the light microscopic level and are largely devoid of the ability to contract.

Prior to the 1990s, treatment of denervated muscle with electrical stimulation was controversial in the UK – in some quarters, it probably still is. At that time, the topic had been studied for maybe 100 years, but the essential characteristics were still not clear.

In the 1960s, *The Denervated Muscle*, edited by Ernest Gutmann, was published, and this work is still not a bad place to start when you wish to learn about this phenomenon (Gutmann, 1962). Gutmann and his collaborators began conducting research on long-term denervation of skeletal muscle in the 1940s and their work is widely cited to this day. Of course, this research is largely descriptive and was limited by the technology available at the time.

It is perhaps still generally believed that no effective treatment is available for muscles that have undergone severe atrophy because of a long-standing denervation injury, but the European research project and multi-national multi-centre study RISE (Kern et al 2010) and work by Helmut Kern and many colleagues and collaborators (Kern et al, 1999) have shown that it is both safe and effective to use a special form of electrical stimulation to rescue muscle tissue bulk and quality with permanently denervated muscles in paraplegic patients. I now have many clients who use this special form of electrical muscle stimulation to manage this situation at home with great effectiveness.

Although I do not expect true functional recovery with complete denervation injuries, there is still a strong reason to persist with electrical stimulation for long-term health. On occasion, I discover injuries are not actually complete and clients recover function they didn't expect to find – it's not a miracle, just that the injury was capable of re-innervation after all. Remember the case of Mark Pollock? He was initially advised that he could not use FES, but he persisted with it and his body responded after some months.

One of the questions I get asked from time to time is: can electrical stimulation damage the possibility of re-innervation? Kern's research concluded that in some people, re-innervation occurs more quickly thanks to this form of stimulation (Kern et al, 1999). In his opinion, nerve regrowth is not inhibited, and this in fact reflects my experience.

It is usually straightforward to produce a muscle contraction with denervated muscle, but special equipment is needed. Commonly available FES units produce waveforms with characteristics that rely on the presence of an intact nerve structure within the muscle, so these will not work when a muscle is denervated. With denervated muscle, we are not looking to activate distinct muscles, but cover as much of a muscle group as possible with a larger form of electrode than that used for FES and have an impact on the muscle structure and its excitability.

Based on the RISE study protocols and extensive research since that time, my business will induce direct contraction of muscle fibres typically by using bipolar rectangular waveforms delivered in shaped bursts and with pulse widths in milliseconds (as much as 150–200 ms rather than the 350–500 microsecond pulse widths used for FES cycling). In addition, it is quite possible that relatively high currents – up to 250 mA – will be required to produce a muscle contraction.

My practical experience and widely available research show that muscle bulk and tissue quality can be restored by this type of stimulation. Large carbon rubber/wet sponge electrodes cover as much of the affected muscle as possible; the gel-type electrodes typically used for FES cycling cannot be used in this situation as the current density applied across the surface of these electrodes would potentially not be tolerated by the skin.

A twitch protocol first improves the excitability of skeletal muscle and its microstructure, and then a tetanic protocol strengthens that muscle. The emphasis in the early days may be on the twitch protocols, and then I would shift to the tetanic approach as the stimulation progresses.

One of the reasons that FES for complete denervation injuries has been controversial in the past is concern about safety. Would skin burns be caused by the high levels of energy required to produce a contraction? Certainly, the levels of current can be higher than those generally considered acceptable for FES applications and different forms of electrodes are needed, but if care is taken, the risk of skin injury is low, so this is safe for home use. This approach still doesn't seem to be as well known as it could be, though, considering its efficacy.

KEY POINT

Stimulation builds muscle, which has aesthetic benefits that users care about as well as reducing pressure ulcer risk and improving local circulation. Stimulate those glutes, not just the muscles we all see.

Electrotherapy and pain

Pain is a big problem for society that health services struggle to deal with. It is not just one thing; pain is complex and can have both physical and emotional components.

The so-called TENS units for pain are widely available and of low cost, but several forms of electrical stimulation can also be used for the symptomatic control of pain. Although the idea had been proposed for many years (decades even), the rationale boost was provided by the so-called 'gate control theory' of pain in the mid-1960s (Melzack and Wall, 1965). Almost certainly, the theory is an oversimplification and the mechanisms of pain generation and perception are being revised and updated all the time, so I won't review them here. I don't find many clients who care too much about a theory – they care about whether something is safe and effective.

Electrotherapy is certainly worth trying for pain relief in many cases as it represents a low-risk intervention and can sometimes be dramatically effective. I tend to get clients who have tried other approaches without success, so have set the bar high anyway. Although it is easy to find so-called TENS machines online that promise to deal with pain at modest cost, in my experience, it may not be clear exactly what type of stimulation these products develop. You may be fortunate and find relief, but it is just as likely that you won't.

Because there is not just one type of pain, there's not one electrotherapy approach, so it takes time and effort to explore the options. Acute pain, which might be referred to by clinicians as nociceptive pain, is closely associated with tissue damage. The body contains specialised nerve cells called nociceptors that detect any noxious stimuli or things that could damage the body, such as extreme heat or cold, pressure, pinching and chemicals. They then pass warning signals along the nervous system to the brain, resulting in our perception of nociceptive pain. As it usually develops in response to a specific traumatic injury situation, nociceptive pain tends to go away as the affected body part heals. For example, pain due to a broken ankle gets better as the ankle heals.

Chronic pain is defined by its persistence for at least three months after healing is presumed to have

TECHNOLOGY

occurred. Neuropathic pain describes the pain that develops when the nervous system is damaged or not working properly due to disease or injury. It is different from nociceptive pain because it does not develop in response to any specific stimulus or trauma. In fact, individuals can suffer from neuropathic pain even when the aching or injured body part is not actually there.

This condition, called phantom limb pain, may occur in people after they have had a limb amputation. It is also relevant to diabetic foot disease and some other forms of nerve trauma following a spinal cord injury. Neuropathic pain may be referred to as nerve pain and is usually chronic.

Electrotherapy products are available that support several waveform types for application across the spectrum of pain manifestations. The ideal product for the professional will allow them to try many approaches with a particular case. Certain waveforms may be favoured in some parts of the world and virtually unknown in others. If this topic is relevant to you, contact me via the details in 'The Author' page and I will point you to more information.

KEY POINT

Electrotherapy can sometimes be dramatically effective for pain relief. Although it is easy to find so-called TENS machines that promise to deal with pain, it may not be clear exactly what type of stimulation they develop.

Transcutaneous spinal cord stimulation

Research has demonstrated that animals with completely severed spinal cords could walk proficiently on a treadmill with partial body weight support (Forssberg, 1980a and 1980b). The theory behind this research, which relied on the presence of so-called central pattern generators, was that the movement of the legs by the treadmill would activate sensory afferents in the limbs that in turn switched on these spinal generators.

This research then explored several non-invasive forms of stimulus energy, such as electrical, magnetic and vibration, and found that they may augment the effects of treadmill training. In this section, we will look at one approach referred to as transcutaneous spinal cord stimulation (TSCS). This approach has been shown since 1982 to enhance the excitability of spinal neural circuits, which has the potential to improve voluntary performance in people with incomplete injuries (Martin, 2021). This research suggests that this change in excitability enables the brain to utilise functionally silent descending pathways to produce and enhance voluntary movements. In other words, it facilitates neuroplasticity.

It is now thought that the priming of the nervous system offered via TSCS could augment existing physical rehabilitation interventions. TSCS, both in single sessions and repeated applications, is associated with improved standing postural control, gait kinematics and upper-extremity function. It has also been demonstrated to have an impact on ANS and non-voluntary functions (such as blood pressure regulation and bladder function). A review looked at the topic in detail for lower-limb and upper-limb applications (Martin, 2021).

Electrical stimulation for the lower limbs is typically delivered with skin surface electrodes placed in accordance with the goals of the exercise. This is done with electrodes over the T11/T12 or L1/L2 intervertebral space and anodes over the iliac crest for the lower limbs. For the upper limbs, a cervical placement is used. A biphasic rectangular waveform of 1 millisecond pulsing with a frequency of 5–50 Hz seems to be typical. Some studies have used a higher frequency carrier signal, but this doesn't seem to be necessary; it appears that a readily available biphasic waveform generator will do the job.

The stimulation current is typically 20–80 mA and adjusted until the participant reports tingling in their extremities. Once the parameters are set, the participant can carry out the activity-based training.

There is a general lack of consensus on stimulation parameters, which may be one reason why this approach has not had greater clinical deployment up until now. Exclusion criteria are generally the same as with other electrical stimulation applications, including open wounds at the stimulation site, pregnancy, active cancer, presence of a cardiac pacemaker/defibrillator or uncontrolled autonomic dysreflexia.

There are many unknowns in relation to this technique and we do not yet understand if the changes associated with it are long lasting, need to be refreshed from time to time or TSCS should be considered like an orthosis and present all the time. Despite this, the results in support of TSCS are compelling. It is low risk and easy to apply as an adjunct to training methods.

An implantable TSCS device, initially devised to treat chronic pain, has received research interest. This epidural stimulator produces similar results to the external stimulator that appear to persist even when it is turned off. Of course, a surgical implant carries a greater risk than the more conservative TSCS approach, so at this early stage, it may be the latter is the appropriate choice.

KEY POINT

TSCS is associated with improved standing postural control, gait kinematics and upper-extremity function, along with an impact on ANS and non-voluntary functions. Currently, though, there are still a lot of unknowns surrounding this technique.

Assistive technology

Most spinal cord injured people are likely to need some form of assistive technology following their injury. Assistive technology is any equipment, product or software program that is used to maintain or improve the functional capabilities of people with disabilities. It can include tools that aid in communication, activities of daily living like toileting, ambulation, eating and grooming, and electronic aids to daily living to control appliances and technology. It's basically anything that allows a person to work around the difficulties that disability can create.

Assistive technology creates opportunities for people with disabilities to participate more fully in all aspects of life, including work and sport. It increases independence, security and control in home, work, leisure and community environments. This is such a broad area that I would struggle to cover all aspects in this book.

In the UK, a useful starting point is to find a company that is a member of the British Healthcare Trades Association (BHTA). The member companies represent pretty much all aspects of healthcare and assistive technology and are bound to operate with trading standards shaped by a code of practice. They recognise that many of their clients are vulnerable, so the code of practice covers all aspects of their interactions.

Charities such as Aspire can help with assistive technology that involves access to a smartphone, tablet or computer.

KEY POINT

Assistive technology creates opportunities for people with disabilities to participate more fully in all aspects of life. Your best course of action is to contact the BHTA or whatever regulatory body operates in your country.

Summary

We have looked in this chapter at several technology areas relevant to spinal cord injury, most of which I have either practical experience of or confidence in their impact. Overall, there is much to be positive about, but progress in technology can never be fast enough for anyone waiting for an improvement in their quality of life.

The public tends to view technological progress as rapid and accelerating, but some of the topics we have covered are not exactly new to the world and represent a long evolution in which evidence of their value has accumulated. Electrotherapy and electrical stimulation are still emerging, despite the fact that this technique was first used by Duchenne 150 years ago. As a safe and effective technology, it has few equals.

Orthotic devices continue to improve through the adoption of new materials and methods of design and manufacture. We can expect orthotic devices to look more like exoskeletons and vice versa over time.

Unfortunately, economics always prevails over technology, so medical device companies face a difficult task in bringing technology products to the market. This is especially true of products which are new to the world. They must be safe and effective, but establishing this is often challenging.

The government directly or indirectly controls technology, partly through its funding mechanisms and partly through its regulatory policies. In an ideal world, regulatory frameworks would be harmonised

TECHNOLOGY

and apply in all countries, allowing developing companies to operate across borders much more easily. We must do what we can to direct public and political attention to this condition, to the impact it has on people's lives, and seek to establish a cure in our lifetimes.

SEVEN
Research Trends

The frustrating thing about research is how long it takes to be applied in practice. There will always be a need for more research, so we don't want to sit back and wait for a particular stream of research to be completed. The chances are it will take longer than we would like, so we must do what we can with what we have right now.

There are no definitive treatments yet for spinal cord injury. Of course, a cure is the aim and research is ongoing to test new therapies. Drugs to limit injury progression, decompression surgery, nerve-cell transplantation and nerve regeneration, as well as nerve rejuvenation therapies, are potential ways to minimise the effects of spinal cord injury.

The biology of the injured spinal cord is enormously complex, but hope for restoring function after paralysis continues to rise – and for good reason. The Brain Research through Advancing Innovative Neurotechnologies (BRAIN) initiative brings together multiple US federal agencies and private organisations to develop and apply new technologies to understand how complex circuits of nerve cells enable thinking, movement control and perception.

Research funded as part of the BRAIN initiative that has the potential to improve the outlook for spinal cord injury includes:

- Looking at brain circuits to better understand the sensory and motor basis of behaviour

- Next-generation neural prostheses (devices that connect to the nervous system and restore functions lost due to disease or injury)

- Improved brain and spinal cord imaging

- New brain-computer interface devices

Basic spinal cord function research studies how the normal spinal cord develops, processes sensory information, controls movement and generates rhythmic patterns (like walking and breathing). Studies using cells and animal models provide an essential foundation for developing interventions for spinal cord injury. Research on injury mechanisms focuses on what causes immediate harm and on the cascade of helpful and harmful bodily reactions that protect from or contribute to damage in the hours and days

RESEARCH TRENDS

following a spinal cord injury. This includes testing of neuroprotective interventions in laboratory animals.

Current research on spinal cord injury is focused on advancing our understanding of four key principles of spinal cord repair:

- **Neuroprotection** – preventing cell death and protecting surviving nerve cells from further damage. This includes drugs to reduce nerve-cell death and controlled lowering of the body's core temperature to reduce cell and blood vessel damage and improve functional outcome.

- **Repair and regeneration** – encouraging the spinal cord's intrinsic ability to self-repair, stimulating the regrowth of nerve-cell projections (axons) and targeting their connections appropriately. This includes cell transplants, natural growth-promoting substances and bioengineered growth scaffolds that allow axons to bridge across the injury site and rebuild neural circuits.

- **Cell-based therapies** – replacing damaged nerve or support cells with other cell types, including stem cells, to regenerate neuronal growth and create new cell connections.

- **Retraining central nervous system circuits** – this restores body functions and forms new nerve connections and pathways (neuroplasticity) following injury or cell death. Techniques include rehabilitation, electrical stimulation (such as

TSCS), robot-assisted training and brain-computer interface technology that may help with voluntary muscle movement and coordination.

Neural engineering strategies build on decades of research that established the field of neural prostheses. For example, researchers are developing a networked FES system to restore independence through combined implants for hand function, postural control, and bowel and bladder control. This has involved the development of experimental brain-computer interfaces that enable people to control a computer cursor or robotic arm directly from their brains (Johnston et al, 2005).

Let's now have a look at each of the four principles in more detail.

Neuroprotection

In the case of spinal cord injury, the initial damage to cells is followed by a series of biochemical stages or events that often knock out other nerve cells in the area of the injury. One aim of neuroprotection research is to modify these secondary processes, thus saving many cells from damage.

The steroid drug methylprednisolone (MP) was approved in the 1990s as a treatment for acute spinal cord injury. MP is believed to reduce inflammation if people get the drug within eight hours of injury, but the medical community is not entirely sold on its effectiveness. Many neurosurgeons won't recommend it and suggest the steroid dosage actually causes more damage.

Meanwhile, research is underway in many labs around the world to find a better acute treatment. Several drugs look promising, including:

- **Riluzole** – protects nerves from further damage from excess glutamate
- **Cethrin** – reduces the growth of inhibitors
- **Anti-Nogo** – a molecule that promotes spinal cord cell growth by blocking inhibition
- **AC105** – proved to be an effective neuroprotective in animal studies and improves motor function in spinal cord injury and cognitive function in traumatic brain injury when initiated within four hours of injury

Cooling of the spinal cord is another possible acute therapy; hypothermia appears to reduce cell loss. Stem cells have also been considered as an acute therapy.

Over a century ago, Spanish scientist Santiago Ramón y Cajal noted that the ends of axons broken by trauma become swollen into what he called 'dystrophic endballs' and are no longer capable of regeneration. This remained a central issue in recovery of function – there seems to be some sort of barrier or scar that traps the nerve tips in place – but recent studies in several labs have revealed that these endballs can get unstuck using the molecule chondroitinase (nicknamed chase) that breaks down the sugar chains forming the scar.

There has been much work published about the potential for chase, which has helped restore function in paralysed animals. There have been no human trials yet; effective delivery of chondroitinase to the injury site has not been fully worked out.

KEY POINT

Initial damage to cells in spinal cord injury tends to be followed by a series of biochemical stages or events that can knock out other nerve cells. One aim of neuroprotection is to modify these secondary processes.

Repair and regeneration

This is perhaps the toughest of the treatment possibilities. To restore a major degree of sensation and motor control after spinal cord injury, long axons must grow again and connect to precise targets over distances as large as two feet.

These axons cannot regenerate unless their path is cleared of poisons, enriched with vitamins and paved with an attractive roadbed. By blocking inhibitory factors (proteins that stop axon growth in its tracks), adding nutrients and supplying a matrix to grow on, researchers have indeed grown spinal nerves over long distances.

One group of scientists at several labs used a molecular switch to turn on nerve-cell growth after trauma (Chen et al, 2018). Phosphatas and TENsin homolog (PTEN) is a tumour suppressor gene that was discovered by cancer researchers. This gene regulates cell growth, and it has turned out to be a molecular switch for axon growth too. When scientists deleted PTEN in a complete spinal cord injury model, cortical spinal axons – the ones needed for major movement function – regenerated at unprecedented rates.

PTEN is complicated. You can't just get rid of it because it is the brake needed to stop certain kinds of cellular overgrowth (cancer), but there are ways to release it. There's still much work to be done to make this relevant to human spinal cord injuries, but many labs are exploring the PTEN gene and others related to regrowth of nerve cells.

In comparison, the idea of a bridge is conceptually easy – transplanted cells, or perhaps a type of miniature scaffold, fill the damaged area of the cord, thus allowing nerves of the spinal cord to cross through otherwise inhospitable terrain. In 1981, Canadian scientists showed that spinal cord axons could grow long distances using a bridge made of peripheral nerves, proving without doubt that axons will grow if they have the right environment (Aguayo et al, 1981). A variety of techniques has evolved through experiments to create a growth-enhancing environment, including the use of stem cells, nerve cells called olfactory ensheathing glia (OEG) that come from the upper nose and Schwann cells (support cells of peripheral nerves).

Another type of bridge – more like a bypass – stitches a piece of peripheral nerve above and below the area of spinal cord lesion. In experiments, a nerve bypass restored some diaphragm function and breathing in animals with high cervical injuries, and some bladder control in animals with lower injuries. Research teams are hopeful this can one day benefit people.

KEY POINT

To restore a major degree of sensation and motor control after spinal cord injury, long axons must grow again and connect to precise targets. By blocking inhibitory factors, adding nutrients and supplying a matrix to grow on, researchers have succeeded in growing spinal nerves over long distances.

Cell-based therapies

While we may dream that broken or lost spinal cord nerve cells can be replaced by new ones, this has yet to become a reality. At present, cell replacement is not possible as a source of spare parts.

Stem cells from a person's own body or from other sources have been used experimentally to restore function after paralysis. Results have been encouraging, but not because the new cells take on the identity of the lost or damaged ones. Replacements simply seem to offer support and help nurture surviving cells. Stem-cell therapy is considered a drug by many medical regulatory agencies and not necessarily approved in spinal cord injury.

Yamazaki et al (2020) reviewed the state of knowledge with a focus on clinical trials that have used stem cells for treating spinal cord injury. It also pointed to the problems that remain to be solved before we will see routine use of this approach. A great number of studies and clinical trials on the stem-cell treatment of spinal cord injury have been conducted worldwide. Although the results are somewhat promising, the most effective treatment strategies are still to be identified. The fact that trials are moving from academia to company-led research is encouraging.

Clinical trials in several countries have tested the safety and efficacy of OEG cells transplanted into the lesion area of the spinal cord and results have been promising. Meanwhile, the Miami Project to Cure Paralysis has begun a clinical trial for transplanted Schwann cells, which have been shown to encourage the regrowth of axons after spinal cord injury.

Combining Schwann cells with other growth molecules may ultimately be more useful than transplants of Schwann cells alone. For example, a team at the Miami Project found that Schwann cells alone activated nerves to grow into a bridge, but they stopped short of crossing the gap in the injured spinal cord. By adding OEG cells to the Schwann cells, the team got the axons to cross the bridge and enter the spinal cord on the other side of the lesion.

> **KEY POINT**
>
> Research is still ongoing into cell replacement, so it'll be some time before this dream is a reality. Early results of various clinical trials are encouraging, though.

Retraining central nervous system circuits

Almost any treatment to restore function after paralysis will require a physical component to rebuild muscle, build bone and reactivate patterns of movement. Some form of rehabilitation will be needed after function comes back.

It appears certain that activity affects recovery. In 2002, seven years after his supposedly complete C2 injury, Christopher Reeve had regained limited function and sensation. His doctor credited his use of FES, which may have kick-started the repair process, and a programme of passive electrical stimulation, aqua therapy and passive standing. To a limited extent, Christopher also used treadmill training, a type of physical therapy that forces the legs to move in a pattern of walking as the body is suspended in a harness above a moving treadmill.

The theory is that the spinal cord can interpret incoming sensory signals: the cord itself is smart. It can carry out movement commands without brain input. Locomotion is managed by the central pattern generators, which activate the pattern of stepping. Stepping during treadmill training sends sensory information to the pattern generators, reminding the spinal cord how to step.

KEY POINT

Rehabilitation techniques have evolved to the point that exercise and physical activity are an essential component of recovery. For the person with a spinal cord injury, it's best to stay active and always strive for the maximum outcome.

Summary

Naturally, research into something as complex as ways to manage and potentially even restore movement after a spinal cord injury is going to be ongoing and never ending. As a result, we can only work with the evidence we have available at any one time.

Current research on spinal cord injury is focused on advancing our understanding of four key principles: neuroprotection, repair and regeneration, cell-based therapies and retraining the central nervous system circuits. We have covered each of these topics in this chapter and the early indications of research are encouraging. There is still a long way to go, though, so I advise the interested reader to keep abreast of the ongoing research.

Final Thoughts

Some years ago, I had the privilege of collaborating with Brigadier Ian Gardiner in a seminar for business on the topic of 'Succeeding in Chaos'. Ian had served with the 45 Commando Group of the Royal Marines and has written about his experiences in the Falklands and the Dhofar war.

Ian taught me that there are only three types of military operation: adjustable military foul ups, semi-adjustable military foul ups and complete military foul ups. This is not as cynical as you might think, but rather an acceptance that there are so many variables and unknowable issues over which we have little influence. War is chaotic, but this does not mean that there is no point in having a plan. There is always a need to know what the mission is and for everyone involved to revise and update the planning as events unfold.

Getting your life back on track after a spinal cord injury is likely to feel chaotic too at times. This does not mean that you should just accept being swept along by events where others dictate every aspect of your life. People may clamour for you to accept the limitations of your condition so that you can move on with your life. You may embrace this and that's fine, but you may not want to accept these limitations. In my view, that is OK too, providing you have a mission and a realistic plan.

First understand your condition in detail and its apparent consequences. This self-knowledge will allow you to have authentic goals that you can believe in. Remember that almost certainly, even a so-called complete injury does not mean that your spinal cord is completely severed. You are unique, so although you might well be given an ASIA score, this does not mean you are identical to other people with the same score. More than this, your circumstances, attitudes, beliefs and expectations will be unique too.

You will need to learn to be your own best advocate and reach out and identify other people and resources that can help you plan, and then achieve your goals. Seek guidance from like-minded people. If people know why you are doing something and how it fits into the bigger picture, they can use their brains and experience to help make it work for you.

I have spent quite a bit of time looking at attitudes and beliefs. In many areas of life, these are the secret sauce that separates success from failure. Reflecting on how you respond to stress and learning to access the most resourceful state that you can is vital to making good choices. Your mindset determines the behaviours that are possible for you, and your consistent behaviours take you step by step to your goals.

Rehabilitation is about recovering as much function as possible (restitution), and then compensating for what you cannot recover. As we humans learn more about neuroplasticity, useful restitution has become a possibility for many more people, and every day, advances are being made, but it's a path with pitfalls. It's best to think about rehabilitation as a journey that needs a training plan and the guidance of others who have been there and done that.

At times, to keep motivated, you will need to focus on the effort rather than the goal and seek a sense of purpose by taking joy from wherever you can find it. Listen to many and varied voices before making a move.

Next moves

I have put together some bonus materials that expand on some of the content I didn't have room for in the book. You can check these out at the website for the book: https://sci-book.anatomicalconcepts.com.

We have an online community for UK clients you can access via our website at anatomicalconcepts.com. Or you can ask me questions via a dedicated email address at book@anatomicalconcepts.com.

Glossary

Abduction – lateral movement of a body part away from the centre of the body.

Adduction – movement towards the centre of the body.

Afferent – conveying impulses from the periphery (arms and legs) towards the central nervous system.

ASIA score – the American Spinal Injury Association classification of spinal cord injuries.

Autophagy – the body's way of cleaning out damaged cells to regenerate newer, healthier cells. This is a natural process necessary for good health.

Axon – a thin fibre that extends from a neuron or nerve cell and is responsible for transmitting electrical signals to help with sensory perception and movement.

Contracture – a limitation in position of a limb joint. For example, a knee flexion contracture means that the knee joint will not fully extend to a normal position.

Denervation – no intact connection between a muscle and the brain. It can occur due to direct injury to a peripheral nerve or by injury to lower sections of the spinal cord.

Disuse atrophy – a loss of muscle tissue and function due to lack of use. It's the body's 'use it or lose it' principle at work.

Electrotherapy – the use of electrical energy as a medical or rehabilitation treatment. In medicine, the term electrotherapy can apply to a variety of treatments.

Excitotoxicity – nerve cells being damaged or dying due to neurotransmitters that are usually both essential and safe reaching pathologically high

GLOSSARY

levels. This leads to receptors being stimulated to excess.

FES – functional electrical stimulation.

FES cycling – combines an FES unit and a passive/active bike or movement trainer. This allows a person with paralysed limbs to exercise their own muscles by synchronising the movement of the bike pedals with delivery of stimulation to these muscles.

Free radicals – oxygen-containing molecules with an uneven number of electrons, which allows them to easily react with other molecules.

Glial scarring (gliosis) – a reactive cellular process involving astrogliosis (a defence mechanism to minimise damage) that occurs after injury to the central nervous system. As with scarring in other organs and tissues, the glial scar is the body's mechanism to protect and begin the healing process.

Hormesis – a principle that recognises that a biological system can adapt to a small amount of stress and become more resilient to a larger amount of stress.

Homeostasis – any self-regulating process by which an organism tends to maintain stability while adjusting to conditions that are best for its survival.

Innervation – an intact connection between a muscle and the brain.

Ischemia – restriction of blood flow, and as a result oxygen, to an area of the body, resulting in local cell and tissue death.

mTOR – stands for the mechanistic target of rapamycin and is a protein kinase regulating cell growth, survival, metabolism and immunity. mTOR is the major regulator of growth in animals and controls most anabolic and catabolic processes.

Myelin sheath – a fatty layer that insulates the axon and helps it transmit signals.

Neuroplasticity – a general umbrella term that refers to the brain and nervous system's ability to modify, change and adapt both structure and function throughout life and in response to experience.

Orthosis – a mechanical structure added to the body to provide support or control a joint range of motion. Orthoses are sometimes referred to as splints or braces. Some simple orthoses may be available off the shelf in a range of sizes and others may be custom made for each individual.

Oxidation – large chemical chain reactions in your body caused by free radicals. They can be beneficial or harmful.

Oxidative stress – an imbalance between free radicals and antioxidants in your body.

Psychophysiology – the study of the mind and body working together as a system.

Rehabilitation – care that can help you get back, keep or improve abilities that you need for daily life. These abilities may be physical, mental and/or cognitive (such as aspects of memory, thinking and learning). You may have lost some ability because of a disease or a spinal cord injury, or as a side effect from a medical treatment.

Restitution – recovering a body function to the level it was prior to injury.

Rhizotomy – a minimally invasive surgical procedure to remove sensation from a painful nerve by killing nerve fibres responsible for sending pain signals to the brain. The nerve fibres can be destroyed by severing them with a surgical instrument or burning them with a chemical or electrical current.

Spasticity – an increased muscle tension with increased muscular proprioceptive reflex.

Transcutaneous spinal cord stimulation (TSCS) – a method of electrical stimulation shown to enhance the excitability of spinal neural circuits. Research is combining this with various forms of activity-based interventions to enhance rehabilitation outcomes.

Bibliography

Abboud, L (2004) 'Drug makers seek to bar "placebo responders" from trials', *Wall St Journal Eastern edition*, 18 June, www.wsj.com/articles/SB108750460497740484

Aguayo, AJ; David, S; Bray, GM (1981) 'Influences of the glial environment on the elongation of axons after injury: transplantation studies in adult rodents', *The Journal of Experimental Biology*, 95: pp231–240

American Spinal Injury Association (1982) *Standards for Neurological Classification of Spinal Injury Patients*. American Spinal Injury Association (ASIA)

Armour, JA (1991) 'Intrinsic cardiac neurons', *Journal of Cardiovascular Electrophysiology*, 2 (4), August, pp331–341

Association of Personal Injury Lawyers (APIL), www.apil.org.uk

Bandler, R (1993) *Time for a Change*. Meta Publications

Barbeau, H; Ladouceur, M; Mirbagheri, MM; Kearney, RE (2002) 'The effect of locomotor training combined with functional electrical stimulation in chronic spinal cord injured subjects: Walking and reflex studies', *Brain Research Reviews*, 40 (1–3), pp274–291, www.researchgate.net/publication/10897466

Benton, B; Iruthayarajah, J; Longval, M; McIntyre, A; Blackport, D; Muise, S; Teasell, R (2019) 'Nutrition issues following spinal cord injury', *Spinal Cord Injury Rehabilitation Evidence*, 7, pp1–69

Buchholz, AC; McGillivray, CF; Pencharz, PB (2003) 'Differences in resting metabolic rate between paraplegic and able-bodied subjects are explained by differences in body composition', *American Journal of Clinical Nutrition*, 77: pp371– 378

Campbell, J (1949) *The Hero with a Thousand Faces*. Princeton University Press

BIBLIOGRAPHY

Chen, C-Y; Chen, J; He, L; Stiles, BL (2018) 'PTEN: Tumor suppressor and metabolic regulator', *Frontiers in Endocrinology*, 9 (July), www.frontiersin.org/articles/10.3389/fendo.2018.00338/full

Claxton, G (2015) *Intelligence in the Flesh: Why your mind needs your body much more than it thinks.* Yale University Press

Clement, JW; Loberg, K (2019) *The Switch: Activate your metabolism for a healthier life.* Simon & Schuster

Cunningham, KJ (2017) *The Road Less Stupid: Advice from the Chairman of the Board.* Keys to the Vault

de la Fuente-Fernandez, R; Schulzer, M; Stoessl, AJ (2002) 'The placebo effect in neurological disorders', Reviews, *The Lancet Neurology*, 1, pp85–91

de la Fuente-Fernandez, R; Ruth, TJ; Sossi, V; Schulzer, M; Calne, DB; Stoessl AJ (2001) 'Expectation and dopamine release: Mechanism of the placebo effect in Parkinson's disease', *Science*, 293, pp1, 164–1, 166

Ditunno, PL; Patrick, M; Stineman, M; Ditunno, JF (2008) 'Who wants to walk? Preferences for recovery after SCI: A longitudinal and cross-sectional study', *Spinal Cord*, 46, pp500–506

DeVivo, MJ; Chen, Y, (2011) 'Trends in new injuries, prevalent cases, and ageing with spinal cord injury', *The Archives of Physical Medicine and Rehabilitation*, 92, pp332–338

Doidge, N (2008) *The Brain that Changes Itself: Stories of personal triumph from the frontiers of brain science.* Penguin

Dong, P; Raffill, T (1996) *Empty Force: The ultimate martial art. The power of Chi for self-defense and energy healing.* Element Books

Duchenne, G; Tibbets, H (1871) *A Treatise on Localized Electrization and its Applications to Pathology and Therapeutics.* Hardwicke

English, J (no date) 'About – Quad-Rebuild', www.quad-rebuild.co.uk/about

Field-Fote, EC; Tepavac, D (2002) 'Improved intra-limb coordination in people with incomplete spinal cord injury following training with body weight support and electrical stimulation', *Physical Therapy*, 82, pp707–715

Forssberg, H (1980a) 'The locomotion of the low spinal cat I. Coordination within a hindlimb', *Acta Physiologica Scandinavica*, 108, pp269–281

Forssberg, H (1980b) 'The locomotion of the low spinal cat II. Interlimb coordination', *Acta Physiologica Scandinavica*, 108, pp283–295

Frankel, HL et al (1969) 'The value of postural reduction in the initial management of closed injuries of the spine with paraplegia and tetraplegia', *Paraplegia*, 7, pp179–192

Gallwey, T (2000) *The Inner Game of Work: Overcoming mental obstacles for maximum performance*. Orion Business

Ginnis et al (2018) 'Evidence-based scientific exercise guidelines for adults with spinal cord injury: An update and a new guideline', *Spinal Cord*, 56, pp308–321

Grillner, S et al (1998) 'Intrinsic function of a neuronal network: A vertebrate central pattern generator', *Brain Research Review*, 26, pp184–197

Gutmann, E (1962) *The Denervated Muscle*. Publishing House of the Czechoslovak Academy, Prague

Guttmann, L (1945) 'New hope for spinal cord sufferers', *Medical Times*, pp318–326

Helms, E; Morgan, A; Valdez, AM (2019) *The Muscle and Strength Pyramid: Training*. Independently published

Hofmekler, O (2017) *The 7 Principles of Stress: Extend life, stay fit and ward off fat*. North Atlantic Books

Irvine, WB (2009) *A Guide to the Good Life: The ancient art of Stoic joy*. Oxford University Press USA

Ivanenko, YP; Grasso, R; Lacquaniti, F (2000) 'Influence of leg muscle vibration on human walking', *Neurophysiology*, 84, pp1,737–1,747

Iyer, MB; Schleper, N; Wassermann, EM (2003) 'Priming stimulation enhances the depressant effect of low-frequency repetitive transcranial magnetic stimulation', *Neuroscience*, 23, pp10,867–10,872

James, W (1948) 'What is emotion'. In: W Dennis (Ed) *Readings in the History of Psychology*. Appleton-Century-Crofts, pp290–303, https://doi.org/10.1037/11304-033

Janssen, T; Glaser, R; Shuster, D (1998) 'Clinical efficacy of electrical stimulation exercise training: Effects on health, fitness, and function', *Topics in Spinal Cord Injury Rehabilitation*, 3 (3), pp33–49

Johnston, TE, et al (2005) 'Implantable FES system for upright mobility and bladder and bowel function for individuals with spinal cord injury,' *Spinal Cord*, 43 (12), pp713–723

Kandel, E; Koster, J; Mack, S; Siegelbaum, S (2013) *Principles of Neural Science* (fifth edition). McGraw-Hill

Kaptchuk, TJ; Miller, FG (2015) 'Placebo effects in medicine', *The New England Journal of Medicine*, 373 (1), pp8–9

Kern, H; Hofer, C; Strohhofer, M; Mayr, W; Richter, W; Stor, H (1999) 'Standing up with denervated muscles in humans using functional electrical stimulation', *Artificial Organs*, 23 (5), pp447–52

Kern et al (2010) 'Home-based functional electrical stimulation rescues permanently denervated muscles in paraplegic patients with complete lower motor neuron lesion', *Neurorehabilitation and Neural Repair*, 24 (8), pp709–721

Kirk, HW (2016) 'Changing the paradigm from neurochemical to neuroelectrical models'. In: *Restoring the Brain: Neurofeedback as an integrative approach to health*. CRC Press

Kirsch, I; Sapirstein, G (1998) 'Listening to Prozac but hearing placebo: A meta-analysis of antidepressant medication', *Prevention & Treatment*, 1 (2), Article 2a

Kohler, R (2010) 'Nicolas Andry de Bois-Regard (Lyon 1658-Paris 1742): the inventor of the word

"orthopaedics" and the father of parasitology',
Journal of Children's Orthopaedics, 4 (4), pp349–355

Lam, K-C (1991) *The Way of Energy: Mastering the Chinese art of internal strength with Chi Kung exercise.* Gaia Books

Langheld, V (2013) *How to Make and Fake Happiness.* Wassermann Publications

Lomas, C (2014) *Finding My Feet.* Claire Lomas Books

Lomas, C (2022) *The Bigger Picture.* Claire Lomas Books

Loughborough University and University of British Columbia (2017) *Scientific Exercise Guidelines for Adults with Spinal Cord Injuries.* Published in collaboration with the National Centre for Sport and Exercise Medicine and the Rick Hansen Institute

Martin, R (2021) 'Utility and feasibility of transcutaneous spinal cord stimulation for patients with incomplete SCI in therapeutic settings: A review of topic', *Frontiers in Rehabilitation Sciences*, 2, www.frontiersin.org/articles/10.3389/fresc.2021.724003/full

Magness, S (2022) *Do hard things: Why we get resilience wrong and the surprising science of real toughness.* Harper Collins

BIBLIOGRAPHY

MASCIP (2013) *Clinical Guideline for Standing Adults Following Spinal Cord Injury*. Spinal Cord Injury Centre Physiotherapy Lead Clinicians United Kingdom and Ireland

McDaid, D; Park, A-La; Gall, A; Purcell, M; Bacon, M (2019) 'Understanding and modelling the economic impact of spinal cord injuries in the United Kingdom', *Spinal Cord*, 57, pp778–788

Melzack, R; Wall, PD (1965) 'Pain mechanisms: A new theory', *Science*, 150, pp971–979

Mitchell, SW (1877) *Fat and Blood: And how to make them*. Lippincott

Mohr, T; Andersen, JL; Biering-Sorensen, F; Galbo, H; Bangsbo, J; Wagner, A; Kjaer, M (1997) 'Long term adaptation to electrically induced cycle training in severe spinal cord individuals', *Spinal Cord*, 35, pp1–16

Mohr, T; Podenphant, J; Biering-Sorensen, F; Galbo, H; Thamsborg, G; Kjaer, M (1997) 'Increased bone mineral density after prolonged electrically induced cycle training of paralyzed limbs in spinal cord injured man', *Calcified Tissue International*, 61 (19), pp22–25

Musselman, K (2007) 'Clinical significance testing in rehabilitation research: What why and how?', *Physical Therapy Reviews*, 12 (4), pp287–296

Ness, LL; Field-Fote, EC (2009) 'Whole-body vibration improves walking function in individuals with spinal cord injury: A pilot study,' *Gait Posture*, 30 (4), pp436–440

NICE (2016) *Spinal Injury: Assessment and initial management* (Clinical guideline). National Institute for Health and Care Excellence, www.nice.org.uk/guidance/ng41

NSCISB (2012) *The Initial Management of Adults with Spinal Cord Injuries*. National Spinal Cord Injury Strategy Board

Paddison, S (1998) *The Hidden Power of the Heart: Discovering an unlimited source of intelligence* (second edition). Planetary Publications

Paleg, G; Livingstone, R (2015) 'Systematic review and clinical recommendations for dosage of supported home-based standing programs for adults with stroke, spinal cord injury and other neurological conditions', *BMC Musculoskeletal Disorder*, 16 (358), https://doi.org/10.1186/s12891-015-0813-x

Pattison, FLM (1986) 'The Clydesdale Experiments: An early attempt at resuscitation', *Scottish Medical Journal*, 31, pp50–52

Pert, C (1997) *Molecules of Emotion: Why you feel the way you feel*. Simon & Schuster

Petrofsky, J; Phillips, C; Heaton, H; Glaser, R (1984) 'Bicycle ergometer for paralyzed muscle', *Journal of Clinical Engineering*, 9, pp13–19, https://journals.lww.com/jcejournal/abstract/1984/01000/bicycle_ergometer_for_paralyzed_muscle.3.aspx

QENSIU (2021) *Queen Elizabeth National Spinal Injuries Unit, Annual Report 2021*. NHS Greater Glasgow and Clyde

Quick, JC, et al (1994) 'Walter Bradford Cannon: Pioneer of stress research', *International Journal of Stress Management*, 1, pp141–143, https://doi.org/10.1007/BF01857607

Robertson, V; Ward, A; Low, J; Reed, A (2006) *Electrotherapy Explained: Principles and practice*. Elsevier Health Sciences

Rowland, JW; Hawryluk, GWJ; Kwon, B, Fehlings, MG (2008) 'Current status of acute spinal cord injury pathophysiology and emerging therapies: Promise on the horizon', *Neurosurgical Focus*, 25, E2

Sallis, RE (2009) 'Exercise is medicine and physicians need to prescribe it!', *British Journal of Sports Medicine*, 43 (1), https://bjsm.bmj.com/content/43/1/3

Salzgeber, J (2019) *The Little Book of Stoicism: Timeless wisdom to gain resilience, confidence, and calmness*. Jonas Salzgeber

Scientific American (2018) *The Science of Diet and Exercise*. Scientific American

SCI Annual Statement (2019) *Specialised Spinal Cord Injury Services Annual Statement 2018/19*. NHS England

SCIRE (2019) 'Nutritional issues following spinal cord injury', *Spinal Cord Injury Rehabilitation Evidence*, Version 7.0, www.scireproject.com (See Benton et al, 2019)

Silver, JR (2003) *History of the Treatment of Spinal Injuries*. Springer Science

Smith, B; Sparkes, AC (2004) 'Men, sport, and spinal cord injury: An analysis of metaphors and narrative types', *Disability & Society*, 19 (6)

Stockdale, JB (1993) *Courage Under Fire: Testing Epictetus's doctrines in a laboratory of human behaviour*. Hoover Institution Press

Stringer, WW; Rossiter, HB (2017) 'Hormesis, mithridatism and Paracelsus: A little oxidative stress goes a long way', *Hypertension Research*, 40, pp29–30

Suez, J et al (2014) 'Artificial sweeteners induce glucose intolerance by altering the gut microbiota', *Nature*, 514 (7521), pp181–186

Thijs, M et al (2016) 'Exercise at the extremes', *Journal of the American College of Cardiology*, 67 (3)

Topol, E (2012) *The Creative Destruction of Medicine: How the digital revolution will create better health care.* Basic Books

Ure, Andrew (1819) 'An account of some experiments made on the body of a criminal immediately after execution, with physiological and practical observations', *Journal of Science and the Arts*, 6, pp283–294

van der Scheer, J et al (2021) 'Functional electrical stimulation cycling exercise after spinal cord injury: A systematic review of health and fitness-related outcomes', *Journal of NeuroEngineering and Rehabilitation*, 18 (99), https://doi.org/10.1186/s12984-021-00882-8

Vawda, R; Fehlings, MG (2013) 'Mesenchymal cells in the treatment of spinal cord injury: current & future perspectives', *Current Stem Cell Research Therapy*, 8 (1), pp25–38

Wade, DT (2009) 'Goal setting in rehabilitation: An overview of what, who and how', *Clinical Rehabilitation* 23 (4), pp291–5, https://doi.org/10.1177/0269215509103551

Wade, DT (2020) 'What is rehabilitation? An empirical investigation leading to an evidence-based description', *Clinical Rehabilitation*, 34 (5), pp 571–583, https://doi.org/10.1177/0269215520905112

Wagner, FB et al (2018) 'Targeted neurotechnology restores walking in humans with spinal cord injury', *Nature*, 563 (7729), pp65–71

Walach, H (2011) 'Placebo controls: Historical, methodological and general aspects', *Philosophical Transactions of the Royal Society B*, 366, pp1870–1878

Wallace, L (2014) 'Indifference is a power', *Aeon*, https://aeon.co/essays/why-stoicism-is-one-of-the-best-mind-hacks-ever-devised

Watson-Jones, R (1955) *Fractures and Joint Injuries* (fourth edition). E & S Livingstone Ltd

Witty, A (2011) 'Research & develop', *The Economist* (22 November), www.economist.com/node/17493432

Wood, J et al (2019) 'Reducing pressure ulcers across multiple care settings using a collaborative approach', *BMJ Open Quality*, 8 (3), https://bmjopenquality.bmj.com/content/8/3/e000409

Yamazaki K, et al (2020) 'Clinical trials of stem cell treatment for spinal cord injury', *International Journal of Molecular Sciences*, 21 (11), p3994

Organisations

Aspire is a charity that provides practical support to people who have been paralysed by spinal cord injury, helping them move from injury to independence. Aspire exists because there is currently no cure. Services include grants, accessible housing, independent living, welfare benefits advice, assistive technology, campaigning and research. For more information, visit www.aspire.org.uk.

Spinal Injuries Association (SIA) is a national user-led charity for spinal cord injured people. It understands the everyday needs of living with a spinal cord injury and meets those needs by providing services to share information and experience and campaigning for change, ensuring each person can lead a full and active life. For more information, visit www.spinal.co.uk.

Back Up is a national charity that inspires people affected by spinal cord injury to get the most out of life. Each year, it reaches over 1,000 people with its award-winning services that are designed and delivered by people affected by spinal cord injury. With a team of over 400 volunteers, the charity offers wheelchair-skills training, an accredited mentoring service, telephone support, life skills and activity courses, and support in returning to work or education. Back Up also offers support to family members and is the only UK charity with dedicated services for children and young people with a spinal cord injury. Find out more at www.backuptrust.org.uk.

Acknowledgements

I experienced a strong sense of imposter syndrome while writing this book. The topic deserves serious attention because a catastrophic injury changes lives. Was I able to do justice to the topic? As a former academic I was used to writing, but this felt different. A book like this was needed, and I only hope that I have made something that is readable and practical. No one can ever be prepared for the consequences of a spinal cord injury, and my personal mission and that of our business is to help people get their lives back on track.

If any of us reflect on past events, we can pick out significant people and places that have steered us this way or that and shaped us to be how we are. I have been blessed with an interesting and challenging career, driven by curiosity and a desire to do more and learn new things. Along the way, I have met many inspirational people, and they are certainly in my mind when I write and work. Acknowledging the individuals below is not intended to diminish the influence of the many clients, carers, healthcare professionals and case managers who have all in one way or another inspired this book.

I originally trained as an engineer and then embraced bioengineering as a different set of challenging engineering problems with a human face. Professor John Paul and 'Bobby' M Kenedi were my first significant and inspirational mentors. They gave us students much scope to work hard and play hard.

Working in Canada, I was privileged to be in the circle of a great set of orthopaedic surgeons. In particular, Bob Salter, Mercer Rang and Norris Carroll were demanding and excellent professionals. It was impossible not to be influenced by their commitment and attention to detail. My home life, too, was enriched by the friendship of my 'second' parents, Doug and Maxine Hartry, and their daughters Nancy, Leslie and Susan.

David Allan, orthopaedic surgeon and then Clinical Director of the Queen Elizabeth National Spinal Injury Unit in Glasgow, connected me to Hasomed GmbH. He nudged me to commit to doing more to improve the lives of those with spinal cord injuries. This led to rich international connections with professional contacts who became friends along the way: the DeToro family, Joe Finocchi, Peter Weber, Andrea Weber and Katrin Bombitzki – thanks for your friendship and support.

ACKNOWLEDGEMENTS

I would like to acknowledge my former partners, Kenneth Munro and William Munro, for their support and friendship in business while we founded and grew Anatomical Concepts.

Andrew Galbraith, of all my professional contacts, has remained a trusted advisor, an inspiration and friend for longer than I dared hope.

I am indebted to Ian Lothian and John Pratt, who introduced me to karate (leaving many bruises), and Michael Breen, who taught me to better understand myself and that the difference between fear and excitement is sometimes just how you breathe.

Finally, thanks to Carolyn Jones, Andrew Galbraith, Claire Lomas, Andy Uttridge, Mark Pollock, Dan Eley, Mark Davies and Mike Ashton for their help in reviewing the first drafts of this book.

The Author

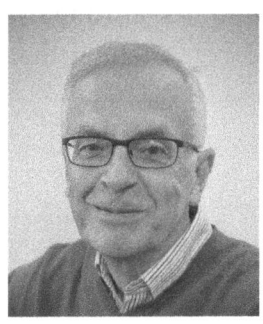Derek Jones's career has involved significant spells in applied research and teaching, followed by entrepreneurship as a business founder and non-executive director. He has always been driven by curiosity and a hunger for knowledge.

Originally trained as a control engineer, he then earned a PhD in bioengineering, followed by scholarships in Switzerland and Canada. His early adventures in rehabilitation were spent in Toronto, Canada with responsibility for developing a research portfolio and a variety of clinical services related to orthopaedics and prosthetics and orthotics.

Returning to an academic career in Scotland, Derek was able to indulge his interest in research and development and innovation in business as he completed his MBA. While serving as a visiting professor at the Cleveland Clinic Foundation, he saw a unique product that eventually led to the creation of Anatomical Concepts (UK) in 1995. He admits to finding it difficult to leave the relative security of academic life to fully commit to business and (dis)credits his MBA studies for teaching him hundreds of ways business can fail.

He has studied NLP with Michael Breen and Richard Bandler and Shotokan Karate to third dan, both of which helped with his personal development and his ever-present fear of failure. Now in his seventh decade, he trains every day he can with the heaviest weights he can and continues an interest in powerlifting and strength and conditioning that started in his teens.

🌐 www.anatomicalconcepts.com

❋ www.linkedin.com/company/anatomical-concepts-uk-ltd

Lightning Source UK Ltd.
Milton Keynes UK
UKHW041440221222
414289UK00004B/143